THE MASCULINE MAN

THE MASCULINE MAN

DAILY LESSONS IN STRENGTH, PURPOSE, AND POWER

DAMIEN RIDER

The Masculine Man

First Edition June 2025
Written and created by Damien Rider

Title: *The Masculine Man*
The Masculine Man: Daily Lessons in Strength, Purpose, and Power
Author: Damien Rider
ISBN: 978-0-6484351-5-0
Cover design by: [Damien Rider]

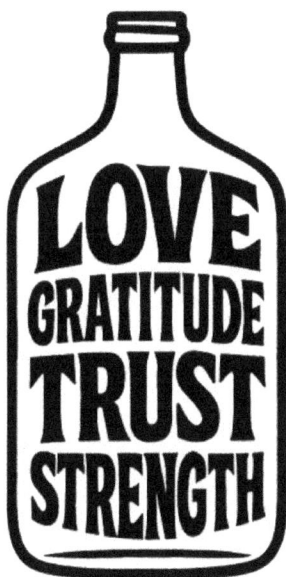

Table of Contents

Introduction

Men, this is your code, with accountable and measured actions to drive your mission, built with strength, purpose, and power to leave your legacy.

This book is the blueprint, not just for how a masculine man thinks, but for how he moves, leads, breathes, dresses, walks, trains, loves, and builds wealth. Discover the code for what it means to be in your complete masculinity in a world that waters men down to their safest, softest versions. It's for the man who feels like he's lost his edge or never found it. It's for the man who knows there's more but doesn't know how to access it.

Now is the moment you stop performing masculinity and start embodying it.
Breath by breath. Day by day. Lesson by lesson.

I've worked with men across all spectrums for over thirty years—world-class athletes, broken fathers, high-level executives, hardened combat veterans, and everyday men carrying an untamed fire inside with no direction. I've seen men built like warriors yet are servants to comfort. Men who have a lot to say but their words carry no weight, Men who follow every rule they were told would make them good yet feel completely lost from who they truly are.

When a masculine man enters a room, the energy shifts because his presence is grounded in discipline, clarity, and something deeper than performance. When he speaks, it's not just heard, it's felt, with every word carrying the strength of purpose. He leads not through dominance, but through embodied service to something greater than himself.

That's who you're here to become.
Not the nice guy—fake, pleasing, passive, invisible.
Not the average man—functioning, drifting, uninspired.
Not just a good man—reliable, loyal, but worn thin.

You're here to become a grounded, dangerous, loving, deeply aware masculine man. The kind of man who can destroy when necessary and nurture without collapsing. The type of man whose discipline is visible, whose boundaries are respected, and whose presence makes people breathe easier, not because he demands it, but because he is it.

When you become that, everything changes. Your body becomes a statement of discipline. Your relationships deepen. You don't chase connection; you create safety through clarity. You don't reach for love; you stand firm in it.

The women in your life don't need saving; they need to feel your grounded presence. Not control, not charm, just steady, masculine energy they can trust. Most have carried the weight for far too long in its absence. They're not looking for perfection. They're waiting for you to become that man—clear, capable, anchored, so they feel it in their nervous system before you ever say a word. Let this book remind you who you are and become the man they remember as someone they can trust.

Over the past decade, I've taken these lessons learned and felt a deep meaning of the words we use, to bottle their layers into something more, for the masculine man.

STRENGTH – Redefining physical and mental endurance.
TRUST – Surrendering to the unknown and letting the mind adapt.
GRATITUDE – Turning suffering into power.
LOVE –Living and leading for something greater than self and guiding others into their transformation daily.

This book helped me sharpen my skills even further as I wrote it. It reminded me that even after all I've done, as men, we are human. We'll make mistakes. We're not perfect. But if we choose to learn, evolve, and lead, we don't just change ourselves. We change the lives of those around us and build a lasting legacy.

A legacy-driven man doesn't chase time; he uses it with precision. He lives fully, teaches what he has earned, and builds what will outlast him. His wealth moves without him. His impact speaks long after he's gone, and he stops asking what he can get and starts asking what will remain because he chose to show up and lead.

Stop trying to be understood and start becoming undeniable.

It's time to remember who you are and start living like it.

Let's begin.

Damien Rider

Athlete Mindset Coach | Wellness Expert | Nature-Based Healer | Founder of OBM & The Evolution Method™

January

Purpose & Accountability

The Foundation of a Masculine Man

You say you want power, impact, and legacy, but without purpose and accountability, those are just empty words. This month isn't here to inspire you, it's here to challenge you. Your life doesn't change when you feel motivated. It changes when you draw the line in the sand and say: "No more drifting. No more blaming. From here on out, I own everything."

Your purpose is defined and clarified through action. Accountability isn't punishment; it's precision. It's the unflinching standard you hold when no one's watching. It's the edge that separates the men who perform strength from the men who embody it.

This month rips off the mask. No sugar coating, no excuses. You will interrogate your values and declare your mission. You will cut out the softness, the hesitation, the vague promises to "do better." You'll start operating like a man who answers only to his highest standard and holds the line no matter the pressure.

A masculine man who's clear on his mission and ruthless with his discipline is the most dangerous, most respected presence in any room. Not with a loud voice. Not because he flexes but because when he speaks, he speaks with purpose, and when he moves, the world feels it.

"A man's life begins the moment he takes full responsibility for it and backs it with purpose."

January 1st

Deep Self-Interrogation

Every man has a foundation buried beneath the noise, and it begins long before adulthood taught him to play roles, chase titles, or follow expectations.

Before the world told you who to be, you acted from instinct, not image. You moved from curiosity, not conformity. That version of you still holds the key to who you are today.

To understand your masculine purpose, you must examine your past, not from nostalgia but from the truth. Sit in silence, remove the distractions, and revisit the earliest moments where you felt fully alive, active, and free. Go back to the activities you did without being told to, like playing with Lego, climbing trees, building bike jumps with friends, doing puzzles, painting, or playing sports. Look at who you naturally were and what gave you joy before the age of 5. The ones that made time vanish as you explored being yourself. Look deeper into why they gave you joy; perhaps it was building something, exploring, leading, problem-solving, creating, or competing. Ask: What drew me to success before anyone told me what it was supposed to look like?

Masculine development starts with this internal view. That's when you ask yourself the question: Am I living a script or a calling? If your current path doesn't align with the essence of who you've always been becoming, you're off course, and the longer you delay, the more that misalignment blocks your power, the longer you feel lost, living in doubt and making poor choices.

The man who reclaims his foundation, who realigns with his origin, doesn't drift; he's grounded and built with clarity, precision, and focus. His accountability isn't a punishment; it's proof that he has a purpose and is living it.

January 2nd

Identify Core Values

A masculine man doesn't change his behaviour based on mood, trends, or approval. He moves from principle, and his strength doesn't come from how loud he roars; it comes from how he knows his code and lives by it. Your purpose isn't something you chase. It's forged in the decisions you make every day based on the values you refuse to break, even when no one is watching.

These values become your edge. They simplify your life. You stop hesitating. You stop negotiating with your soul. You start leading from within, and when darkness falls, you're not guessing who you are; you already know and can move through it with ease.

Action:

1. Strip everything back.
2. Sit in silence. No phone. No distractions. Ask yourself: If I lost every title, every follower, every dollar, what would I still believe in?
3. Write down your non-negotiables.
4. Choose 3 to 5 values that define how you live and lead. Not what sounds good, but what you'd go to war for. Discipline. Truth. Loyalty. Honour. Precision. Choose your code.
5. Test them under fire.

6. Examine your last three difficult decisions. Did you act from those values or abandon them to be liked, safe, or comfortable?

7. Reinforce them daily.

8. Say them out loud each morning. Before making a hard decision, check it. Before you speak, lead, or act, align with your code.

January 3rd

Define Your Mission

Your mission is the anchor that holds you steady when pressure hits and the fire and passion within that pulls you forward when comfort tempts you to slow down. It's not about grandeur or applause. It's about meaning. Impact. Precision. The masculine man operates with direction, and that direction comes from a mission he chooses, defines, and is committed to.

This mission becomes your filter. You'll say no faster. Move bolder. You won't just exist; you'll live with purpose on purpose, and when the fire inside is stronger than the storm outside, you become unstoppable.

Action:

1. Ask the hard question:
2. In silence, write this at the top of a page: What would make all my struggle, pain, and sacrifice worth it?
3. Don't censor. Don't edit. Write what stirs your gut, not what looks good on paper.

   Identify your impact:
4. Who do you want to serve? What problem are you here to solve? What shift will happen in the world, community, or family because you showed up and did the work?

5. Write your mission in one sentence:

6. For example:

   "I use my experience to build high-performing men who lead with power and peace."

7. Test it against resistance:

8. Read it when you're tired in times of doubt. When life kicks you down, if it doesn't move you and feel right, then refine it until it does.

9. Post it somewhere visible:

10. Not on social media. Let it permeate how you train, speak, lead, and present yourself.

January 4th

Purpose Builds Unshakeable Confidence

When a man is grounded in purpose, he no longer needs permission to act or external applause to feel valid. His clarity becomes his armour. He doesn't slow down when facing resistance because his direction is rooted deeper than his fears. Absolute masculine confidence isn't loud; it's unshakable. It's the stillness of a man who knows exactly why he gets up in the morning, who understands what he's building every day, who he is becoming, and what lines he'll never cross.

That kind of man doesn't ask, "Am I good enough?" He asks, "What's my next move?" Purpose removes the fog and mental distortion and cuts through the noise of social expectation and emotional confusion. You stop needing to overexplain yourself. You stop shrinking to make others feel comfortable. You stop flinching when life hits you hard because even if you're battered and bruised, even if you're tired, you know why you're here. Knowing is what makes your presence powerful, and your leadership respected. When a man operates from purpose, confidence isn't something he turns on; it's what he embodies.

January 5th

Purpose Drives Relentless Action

When a man has locked onto a purpose that resonates deeply, not a fantasy or a copy-paste goal, but a visceral reason to live each day, he no longer hesitates. He executes. He doesn't waste time scrolling, second-guessing, or needing constant external motivation and approval. The purpose-driven man doesn't have to convince himself to act; the mission drives him, and when others falter under pressure, he steps in, not because it's easy, but because he knows what's at stake and understands that if he doesn't, who else will?

Purpose gives weight to every action, whether you feel like doing it or not. It's the reason you finish reps after failure, and it's why you keep pushing when comfort would be the easier path. The attitude of grinding through struggle dissolves because a masculine man is building something bigger than ego, something bigger than any wall put in front of you. You're building impact, legacy, and character.

The masculine man becomes unstoppable, not by chasing intensity, but by waking up every day and giving everything to something that truly matters.

Action:

1. Identify Your Why – Write down the one thing you'd still fight for when everything else falls apart. Be honest. If it doesn't stir your gut, go deeper.

2. Set a Daily Anchor – Every morning, revisit that reason. Write it, speak it, or meditate on it for two minutes.

3. Eliminate Half-Commitments – Audit where you're moving without aim. Cut anything that drains energy but doesn't serve your mission.

4. Track Effort, Not Just Outcomes – Keep a record of daily execution, not just wins. The purpose is proven in process, not quick results.

5. Reaffirm During Fatigue – When you feel like quitting, ask: "Does my mission still matter?" If the answer is yes, move. If not, refine it.

January 6th

Explore Pain Points

Every man carries a wound, sometimes so deeply buried that it gets mistaken for personality. The masculine man doesn't shy away from his pain. He turns and faces it head-on. Your purpose shines through in the raw, scarred places where life has tried to break you or has already broken you. That heartbreak, betrayal, abandonment, failure, addiction, whatever shaped the darkness within, holds the key to his edge, empathy, and direction.

When you stop hiding your pain and start examining it, you begin to see how it has sculpted your character. You see the lessons learnt, the emotional strength built under pressure, the values you forged through your inner fire. When you own that, without shame or victimhood, you tap into something far more profound than ego; you touch a mission that's personal, embodied, and bulletproof. That's where the masculine path begins to carve a legacy; through healing comes service, and scars become a source of strength.

You don't become a masculine leader by pretending to be untouched. You become one by transforming your history into fuel and then using it to light the way for others.

Action:

1. Create a Sacred Space – No distractions—just pen, paper, and silence. Sit with yourself and revisit the pain points you've buried.

2. Write Your Battle Wounds – List the top 3 most challenging moments you've faced. For each, write how it changed you, what it taught you, and who it made you become.

3. Find the Common Thread – Look at those events and ask: What patterns show up? What values and gifts were born from this pain?

4. Define Your Message – From those lessons, write one statement that reflects how you can help others with what you've lived through. Begin to reveal your deeper purpose.

5. Transform, Don't Transmit – Decide to use the pain as fuel, not a disguise. Let it sharpen you, not soften you.

January 7th

Build Unshakeable Confidence

A man without a purpose is a man chasing an identity. His confidence rises and falls with the opinions of others, market trends, or his sense of well-being on any given day. When a masculine man is grounded in a clear purpose and living his mission, everything about him changes, not just how he moves but why he moves. Purpose gives his confidence a foundation. It's the difference between performing strength and embodying it. True confidence isn't loud; it's not a puffed-up chest or forced bravado. It's calm, grounded certainty that doesn't flinch, doesn't need to explain itself, and doesn't need applause to know you are walking the right path.

Purpose strips away hesitation. You stop asking, "Should I?" and start acting like a man who has already decided. You become more precise with your energy, less reactive to chaos, and intensely loyal to your standard, not because you're perfect but because you're clear. That clarity, that internal alignment, is where unshakeable confidence thrives.

Confidence comes from knowing exactly who you're and why you're here and backing that up with action.

Action:

1. Write Your Purpose Statement – One sentence. No fluff. Something that makes you stand taller when you read it.

2. Recite It Daily – Before you face the world, face yourself. Read it out loud with conviction.

3. Act in Alignment – Filter your decisions through this question: Does this move serve my mission or distract me from it?

4. Refine Through Fire – Test it. Let life test you. If you hold under pressure, it's real. If you break, go deeper and rewrite.

January 8th

Seek Patterns of Passion

To understand what drives you, you must study the consistent signals your life has sent you, not the noise, not the obligations, but the fire in your belly. The experiences where time vanished, the effort felt effortless, and you moved from an undeniable knowing without needing a reason were driven by your intuition, not accidents. They were markers and indicators of alignment. When you trace them with intention, they start to reveal a map and a pathway of a recurring theme in how you lead, build, compete, serve, or create.

Every man carries this internal compass, but few take the time to read it. Most get swept up by demands, pulled into roles they never chose, and lose sight of what genuinely lights them up. For the masculine man, passion isn't an indulgence; it's information. It's the raw material of purpose. The repeated pull toward specific ideas, actions, or arenas isn't just a matter of preference; it's the design that gives you an edge. Once you know what energises you, you can construct your life around it instead of constantly fighting against your natural flow.

Your purpose isn't something you borrow, mimic, or manufacture. It's the intersection of your deepest curiosities and your highest capacities. If you've always been a leader, that's not just ego; it's a calling. If you've lost hours building things from scratch or strategising how to win, that's not a distraction; that's a signal. If you find meaning when you teach, help, or protect others, then those are not just admirable qualities; they're directional.

The man who walks in alignment with his passion becomes unstoppable, not because life gets easier, but because he finally knows which battles are his to fight.

January 9th

Prioritise Your Time

A man without purpose reacts to life instead of directing it. Your schedule is cluttered with other people's expectations, low-value tasks, and surface-level social obligations that drain your energy and soften your edge. The masculine man understands that time is finite, non-refundable, and sacred. It's not just a calendar entry; it's your life, moment by moment, choice by choice.

If your purpose doesn't fuel your mission, build your body, sharpen your mind, elevate your circle, or expand your legacy, it doesn't make the cut and sets you up for energy depletion. You don't owe anyone your time. You owe yourself your full capacity. That means cutting the excess without guilt, whether that's reducing screen time, keeping people at arm's length, cancelling plans that no longer align, or delegating work that pulls you off course.

Action:

1. Audit Your Calendar — Open your weekly schedule and highlight what builds your mission versus what distracts you from it. Be ruthless.

2. Identify Time Leeches — List the three activities, people, or habits that consume the most time without a measurable return on investment (ROI). These must be reduced or eliminated.

3. Clarify Your Top 3 Priorities — Right Now. Be specific. Example: "Grow my business revenue by 20%," "Build myself to elite-level fitness," "Lead the next generation with strength and presence."

4. Design Your Ideal Week — Allocate protected time blocks daily to those three things. Treat them like non-negotiable, unmissable appointments.

5. Say No Without Apology — Script it if you must: "That doesn't align with where I'm going right now." Say it calmly, firmly, and without guilt.

January 10th

Connect with Impact

The masculine man knows that strength must be shared, not hoarded. He realises that the actual test of his character is not just how high he climbs but who he pulls up as he rises. His journey may start in solitude, but it must end in significance and abundance.

To make an impact, you must look beyond yourself. Ask yourself: Who needs what I've already learned the hard way? Who's struggling in the dark with problems I've already solved? Who could rise faster if I gave them a roadmap or the courage to keep going? Your purpose becomes a legacy when your pain becomes someone else's breakthrough, when your discipline becomes someone else's structure, and when your presence becomes someone else's safety.

It's not about becoming a martyr or a saviour; it's about becoming a man who lives with impact embedded in his decisions, mission, and purpose. Whether it's mentoring young men, protecting your family, leading your team, or guiding a partner, the masculine man operates with the awareness that every move affects those around him. This awareness fuels him on days when motivation has gone. It's not just about him; it's about who needs him to show up fully.

Real masculine purpose is the voice that reminds you that everything you do or put off doing either strengthens or weakens your ability to lead, protect, and provide for those who count on you. A legacy stays alive through sacrifice, discipline, and the consistent decision to live as the person others can depend on.

Action:

1. Who do you feel called to serve?
2. What specific skills, wisdom, or experience do you have that could shorten someone else's suffering?
3. Who would be worse off if you didn't show up in your full strength?

January 11th

Attract the Right People

When you walk with clear direction and unwavering standards, you no longer need to convince people to believe in you. Your actions speak it. Your discipline proves it. Your energy announces it. Your purpose isn't just internal alignment; it's magnetic authority. You don't beg for seats at someone else's table; you build the table, and people want to sit at it. They feel something from you that's rare in this world: certainty and vision.

Ask yourself: If I fully embodied my mission, who would feel compelled to rise beside me? Who would want to join, support, or invest in what I'm building? Purpose cuts through superficial networking and empty relationships. It attracts teammates, mentors, partners, and high-level allies who are drawn not to what you want but to who you've become.

When your mission becomes undeniable, the right people won't need convincing; they'll recognise where they belong.

Action:

1. Write down your core mission in one sentence. No fluff. Make it something you'd be proud to stand on a stage and speak.

2. Audit your inner circle. Who energises you? Who drains you? Who sharpens your edge? Who keeps holding you back?

3. Share your vision out loud. In conversations, on platforms, and your work, let it be known. Stop hiding what drives you.

January 12th

Amplify Influence

In a world full of noise, indecision, and superficial ambition, the man with purpose stands apart. He doesn't have to dominate the room with volume; his presence does the work. People sense when a man knows exactly who he is and what he's building. That clarity becomes contagious. It shifts the emotional temperature in the room, commands attention without force, and earns loyalty without manipulation.

When you live in alignment with your mission, your habits, decisions, and sacrifices reflect a clear internal compass, and other people instinctively trust you. They see you lead yourself, and in that, they trust you to lead others. Influence is earned through consistency, certainty, and sacrifice in service of something bigger than yourself.

Ask yourself: Are my actions proof of my vision? Do I lead with example or expectation? If not, recalibrate and let your mission speak through execution. The masculine man doesn't seek followers; he moves with such focus that others choose to walk beside him.

Key elements to amplify your influence through purpose:

1. Embodiment: You are the first to do the hard thing, not just tell others to do it.

2. Clarity: You can articulate your mission with confidence and clarity.

3. Consistency: People can rely on your presence, your habits, and your standards.

4. Service: You make others better through your pursuit, not just your success.

January 13th

Step Into Challenges

Purpose is built in struggle. Aiming for a life of comfort has never made a man powerful. The masculine man understands that to live with purpose, he must willingly step into the ring because only under pressure can proper direction, grit, and clarity emerge. Your purpose isn't some vision board fantasy or a journaled ideal. It's carved into your bones when you face what most avoid.

Suppose you're serious about being a man of depth and facing consequences. In that case, you must ask yourself: When was the last time I chose a path that demanded more of me, physically, mentally, and emotionally? That's where purpose sharpens, when you're tired, doubting, and stretched, yet still choose to keep moving forward.

A test and a challenge are not the enemy; they're the invitation. Whether it's stepping into uncomfortable conversations, enduring physical pain for a worthy goal, or facing a fear you've suppressed for years, challenge clarifies what matters. It exposes the gap between what you say you want and what you're genuinely committed to. What you fear and avoid is where the lesson lies.

A man's purpose comes alive not when you avoid the tests presented to you but when you realise you are a warrior preparing for war.

Action:

1. Identify one challenge each week that makes your stomach tight, your breath short, your mind race, and face it head-on. It could be physical (running when exhausted), relational (having the conversation you've been avoiding), or professional (pursuing the uncomfortable next step).

2. Reframe hardship as data. Every setback teaches you more about your edge and whether you're committed to your mission.

3. Build a challenge into your lifestyle. Cold exposure, early rising, fasting, training, and long periods of focused work. Use adversity to train your nervous system to stay calm under pressure.

January 14th

Get Feedback

A man's purpose must dominate within, though it often becomes visible externally through the way others respond to him, lean on him, or speak about him when he's not in the room. You may think you know your mission, but you're also living inside your blind spots. That's where feedback becomes essential, not as approval but as clarity.

Every man has gifts he underestimates. Talents you downplay. Patterns of power you don't see because they come so naturally that you assume they're ordinary. What's ordinary to you may be extraordinary to someone else. That's why a man serious about embodying your mission must seek out high-integrity mirrors —people who see you fully and tell you the truth without flattery or sugar coating to protect your feelings.

When multiple people reflect a similar strength or moment of impact, that's not a coincidence. That's your signal. Your purpose is to leave a trail, not just in your passions, but in your impact, often seen more clearly by those you've affected than by yourself.

Be willing to hear the uncomfortable truths, too: where you're playing small or holding back, where your energy leaks and is wasted, and where you show inconsistency. A man committed to purpose welcomes correction, not because you doubt yourself but because you're devoted to sharpening yourself.

The masculine man integrates what others see in you into what you know of yourself and becomes even more lethal in the pursuit of his mission.

Action:

1. 1. Schedule one-on-one conversations with 3-5 trusted people: a mentor, a partner, a teammate, a coach, and a brother. Ask them direct questions about your strengths, blind spots, and moments they've seen you lead with impact.

2. 2. Record and reflect on what's said. Don't argue. Don't explain. Just listen, then look for recurring themes or insights that resonate deeply with you.

3. 3. Use feedback to recalibrate your mission statement. Ask: What part of me am I compelled to amplify, protect, or evolve based on what's reflected?

January 15th

Transform Adversity into Growth

The masculine man doesn't fear adversity; he welcomes it and ultimately transcends it. Hardship, pain, loss, and failure are not the end of the road for a man living with purpose; they are the terrain he was born to traverse.

When adversity strikes, most men collapse into self-pity or stagnation. You stop asking why this is happening to me and instead ask the only question that matters: How can this shape me stronger? A masculine man knows that every hardship contains the seed of power if he's willing to utilise the lesson. When you process pain with clarity and intention, it becomes the next step in your evolution.

To grow through adversity, you need to make a shift from a state of victimhood to one of strategy. You must begin to see every experience, no matter how brutal, as a way that strengthens and benefits you and your purpose. Your most powerful impact often comes from the places you once thought would break you. Whether it's betrayal, bankruptcy, injury, heartbreak, or failure, all of its raw material that you turn into fuel.

Action:

1. Document your pain points from the past five years and the hardest things you've faced. Next to each one, write the lesson it taught you. Ask: What strength did I develop because of this?
2. What skill emerged?
3. Build from the scar, not the wound. Don't just relive the trauma; refine it. Integrate it into your mission by using it to guide others, improve systems, or strengthen your code.
4. Reframe setbacks in real-time. When something goes wrong today, please don't waste time resisting it; instead, focus on resolving the issue. Pause. Breathe. Then, ask, "How is this beneficial for me to adapt and keep moving forward?"

January 16th

Ignites Peak Performance

Purpose is the precise driving force that aligns all systems of a man, activating his mental clarity, physical strength, emotional regulation, and spiritual stamina in unison. His purpose ignites peak performance because it filters distraction and annihilates hesitation. It gives meaning to discomfort and converts resistance into fuel. In the gym, it turns reps into ritual. In business, it transforms stress into strategy. In relationships, it converts presence into power. Every move becomes calculated, intentional, and infused with meaning. You are no longer doing things to succeed; you are doing them because they serve the mission. That depth changes your standard and makes mediocrity feel intolerable.

Peak performance is not about constant speed or effort; it's about alignment. When your actions lock into your highest purpose, you don't burn out chasing ten different things. You channel your energy like a sniper; you recover faster, think clearly, train harder, and perform more precisely because your nervous system, mindset, and habits are all calibrated to a singular mission. That's the true performance edge, not some hack or secret, but a deep-rooted reason to give everything you've got every single time.

January 17th

Own Every Outcome

A masculine man doesn't flinch when outcomes fall short and doesn't wait for someone else to clean up the fallout. You own it with a steel spine and open eyes built on action and ownership. If the plan fails, if you don't achieve the result, or if your team misses the points, examine your role first. The moment you blame anything outside of yourself, you give away your power.

Owning every outcome doesn't mean self-blame or beating yourself up. It means taking full authority over your life, your choices, and your standards. It means asking, "Where did I drop the ball?" "What pattern am I repeating?" "Where was I not clear, not focused, not disciplined?" It's brutal sometimes, but that brutal clarity is what sharpens a man into a leader.

It's how you teach your nervous system that failure is just a moment or an identity. When you own everything, not just your wins but your wounds, you become unstoppable.

Action:

1. Adopt a zero-blame policy. At the end of each day, ask yourself three things:
2. What did I execute with excellence?
3. Where did I fall short?
4. What can I do differently tomorrow to get back on track?

January 18th

Build Ironclad Integrity

Integrity is not a personality trait. It's a commitment built on your actions, tested under pressure, and refined through clear accountability. For the masculine man, integrity is the non-negotiable foundation, the steel backbone that holds everything else upright. Without it, your strength is performative, your leadership is hollow, and your purpose is unstable. Integrity is what separates men who talk about being leaders from those who lead by living their values visibly, consistently, and without excuse.

Living with ironclad integrity means doing what you say, when you say it, and how you say it, especially when no one is watching. It's the courage to speak the hard truth when it would be easier to stay silent. It's showing up on time. It's saying no when your values are on the line, even if it costs you the deal, the relationship, or the applause. Integrity is the daily decision to be accountable to your mission, your word, and your higher standard, regardless of the outcome.

You don't wait for someone else to call you out. You call yourself out. You self-audit. You course correct and you understand that a man who lies to himself has already lost his edge. When your integrity is intact, your power multiplies. Others may not always agree with you, but they'll trust you, and that trust becomes your leverage in business, brotherhood, and love.

Integrity with purpose means your mission isn't just an idea; it's something you bleed into your actions. Every decision aligns with your core values. Every move reflects your code. That alignment becomes your compass when darkness hits. You never need to scramble or panic because you've already chosen who you are and what you stand for.

Integrity with accountability means you don't hide behind excuses, blame, or half-truths. If you are unsuccessful in an attempt, own it. If you broke it, fix it. If you said it, follow through. Masculine strength isn't just about domination; it's about consistently recalibrating for self-mastery.

January 19th

Analyse Without Ego

True masculinity is clear, direct, and grounded in self-awareness, and that means analysing your actions without letting your ego sabotage the truth. When something doesn't go as planned, whether it's a failed conversation, a setback in your business, a missed opportunity, or a moment where your emotions got the better of you, your job as a man isn't to explain it; blame others, or hide behind pride. Your job is to dissect it with surgical precision.

Most men fold, protecting their self-image instead of using it as a means of growth. You don't grow by defending your ego; you grow by killing it in those moments. Masculine maturity starts the moment you stop fooling yourself. You ask the fundamental question: "What part of this did I control?" "What did I ignore that I should've addressed?" "What did I say or do that made this better or worse?" "Where did I let pride overrule precision?"

It isn't a weakness; it is elite-level accountability. When you strip away excuses and emotions, you start to see patterns: where you hesitate, where you act out of fear, and where you default to comfort. That's the information that separates men who repeat their mistakes from men who build power with every setback. This form of analysis is tactical for becoming a better leader, a stronger partner, and a sharper strategist because you're constantly refining your decisions and behaviour.

Action:

1. Tonight, carve out 10 minutes with no distractions and no scrolling. Choose one moment from your day that tested you even slightly. Write down three things:
2. What did I do that moved things forward?
3. What did I avoid or delay that weakened the outcome?
4. Where did pride, defensiveness, or ego show up?

January 20th

Accelerate Growth

Masculine growth grows through intelligent intensity. If you're still relying on willpower alone, you're playing small and holding back. Growth at the highest level doesn't come from grinding harder; it comes from getting more efficient with how you train your body, shape your thoughts, structure your time, and sharpen your emotional responses. A masculine man is committed to his purpose and builds systems that multiply your growth, not just routines that maintain it.

What you feed your mind, your nervous system and your circle will either accelerate you or dilute you and slow your mission. Choose books, mentors, environments, and conversations that widen your perception, not repeat your past. Surround yourself with men who demand your evolution, not your comfort. Audit your information daily and replace draining noise with content that fosters precision thinking, emotional regulation, and strategy.

Measure your sleep, training intensity, nutrition, journaling, and execution of your mission. If you want to grow faster, data is your ally. Train like an elite athlete would: review performance, identify patterns, make corrections for more efficiency, and start to grow with intention.

Integrate recovery as a weapon. Masculine power comes not just from how hard you push but also from how quickly you can reset.

Use Breathwork to regulate your state and to recalibrate stress and emotions. Use Breathwork, like One Breath Meditation or presence drills, to reset your nervous system in under a minute.

Use time-blocking, task-stacking, and decision-elimination strategies. Focus with intensity and finish with precision. Instead of running on adrenaline, learn to run on rhythm. Expand your growth edge weekly with voluntary discomfort, hard physical training, high-stakes communication, and emotional honesty.

The masculine man doesn't hope to grow; you engineer it.

January 21st

Use Failure as Fuel

A masculine man doesn't fear failure; he extracts strength from it. When purpose drives your path, failure serves as a checkpoint, exposing your edges and refining your mission. Most men fold when things fall apart. They retreat into excuses, shame, or paralysis. A man in command studies failure like a tactician, because buried in every misstep, is the exact roadmap to move forward with more precision, more power, and a stronger purpose.

Failure isn't proof you're unworthy. It's proof you're in the arena. The masculine frame understands that every fall is a data point, an insight into a broken system, an outdated mindset, or a weakness. When you face failure without ego, you stop reacting emotionally and start responding strategically. You ask: "What part of me was not yet ready?". Then, breathe, adapt, refine, and rise again.

Turning failure into fuel begins with radical accountability. No blame. There is no drama; just sitting with it in complete ownership. If it falls apart, you take the wheel and rebuild with more force and fewer flaws. This accountability reclaims your internal power, the same power that builds men who finish what they start, no matter the resistance. That's how a mission stays alive, not through perfection but through persistence sharpened by every cut.

Create Unshakeable Confidence

Absolute confidence isn't a performance. It isn't about puffing your chest, speaking louder, or dominating a room. It's the kind that radiates power before you say a word; it comes from a knowing, deep in your bones, that you are a man who follows through. A masculine man earns that knowing through one thing: ownership. Full-spectrum, no-excuse, take-the-wheel ownership of your life, your results, your responses, and your energy.

When you own every outcome, from victories to failures, half-finished projects, and missed marks, something powerful shifts, and you stop waiting for someone to affirm your worth because you know where you stand. You've made decisions, taken hits, gotten back up, and corrected your course. It tells your nervous system, "I've got this. No matter what."

This kind of confidence is evident in the way you move, deliberate, unhurried, and grounded. It sharpens your communication because you're not speaking to impress; you're speaking with clarity and self-trust in your words. It holds you steady in relationships, business, and battle because you don't need control when you have command.

Confidence built on ownership is unshakeable because it doesn't rely on perfect conditions; it's forged in whatever conditions are in front of you; that's how you embody the edge and certainty.

January 23rd

Hold Yourself to a Higher Standard

A man living with purpose doesn't wait for the world to challenge him; he challenges himself. Holding yourself to a higher standard means you reject mediocrity in all its subtle forms: cutting corners, justifying laziness, and tolerating a half-hearted effort. It's about demanding more from yourself because you know what's at stake: your character, your mission, your purpose, and your legacy.

This standard is the unspoken agreement you make with yourself that says, "I do what's required and then more". It becomes the invisible scaffolding that supports every part of your masculine foundation. Whether you're alone in the dark or standing in the spotlight, you hold the same posture, speak the same truth, and deliver the same level of precision and excellence. That consistency creates internal trust, and once you trust yourself, you become untouchable.

It's also how accountability stays alive. You don't feel external pressure when your internal standard is higher than any coach, partner, or boss could ever set, and this is where purpose becomes powerful. When your standard aligns with your mission, every action, every rep, and every decision becomes infused with meaning.

Action:

1. Identify one area of your life, fitness, work, relationships, or mindset where you've been coasting on "good enough."

2. Now, raise the standard. Set a specific rule that reflects your higher self, whether it's waking up earlier, finishing what you start, speaking with greater clarity, or training with absolute focus.

3. For the next 7 days, commit to that rule with zero negotiation. Become the man you're proud to follow.

January 24th

Attract Respect and Leadership

Authentic leadership is earned, quietly and consistently, by the man who leads himself before he tries to lead anyone else. A masculine man rooted in purpose and accountability doesn't need to posture or dominate to gain respect. Your influence comes from how you show up when no one's watching, how you handle failure, how you adjust when off course, and how you stand firm when pressure rises. People are drawn to unshakable men, not because you're perfect, but because you're responsible.

When you own your outcomes, especially the painful ones, and resist the urge to deflect or excuse, you send a clear message: "I can carry the weight". That emotional weight, or that mental pressure, is what separates boys from men. You become the one others look to, not because you bark commands but because you've proven you can take the hit and keep moving with clarity and purpose.

This level of personal responsibility builds magnetic respect, the masculine path where leadership isn't optional; it's inevitable for the man who holds the line when others fold.

Action:

1. Think of one recent mistake or failure, whether personal or professional, that you've avoided talking about or tried to explain away.

2. Call or meet with a trusted peer or mentor or sit with it without judgment and unpack it down to its raw foundation, with full ownership. That act alone sets a standard others will respect.

January 25th

Cut Out the Victim Mentality

A masculine man doesn't live in blame. He refuses to see himself as a casualty of circumstance because he knows that every time he points the finger outward, he weakens his authority. Victimhood is seductive; it gives you a story that justifies inaction, a reason to stay small, and a shield against responsibility. The longer you live in it, the more you convince yourself that life is happening to you instead of being shaped by you.

Real masculine power starts when you cut out the language of powerlessness when you stop saying, "They did this to me", and start asking, "What's the next move I can make?" That shift doesn't erase pain or injustice, but it does put the wheel back in your hands. You're not responsible for everything that happens to you, but you are 100% responsible for how you respond, how you adapt, and how you use the moment to sharpen your edge.

The man who eliminates the victim mindset becomes unshakable because nothing can trap you for long. Setback? You learn from. Betrayal? You rebuild wiser. Loss? You mourn, then move forward. It's not cold detachment; it's sovereign self-command. When you reclaim ownership over your response, you reclaim your life. That's where strength is born, not from control but from accountability.

January 26th

Eliminate Energy Drains

Every time a masculine man complains, points fingers, or ruminates on what someone else did wrong, you're wasting valuable energy to advance your mission. Emotional blame is the costliest tax a man can pay; it robs you of momentum, clouds your clarity, and lowers your frequency. Masculinity isn't just about physical strength; it's about energetic control. It's about guarding your internal resources as fiercely as a warrior defends his camp.

When you shift from blame to ownership, your energy becomes more consolidated. You transition from a scattered reaction to a directed response. Being a masculine man is not about controlling others; it's about mastering yourself. It's about staying entirely in your lane, tracking your choices, tone, timing, and mindset. Even when others act out of alignment, you don't fold. You assess, adapt, and act with purpose.

You don't ignore wrongdoing or bypass pain; you don't give it free rent in your psyche. You don't replay the story of how someone failed you; you write the next chapter based on how you rise. That's the essence of masculine power: cutting emotional clutter, deleting distractions, and transforming every ounce of your energy into forward movement.

Action:

1. Think back to a recent moment where you felt drained, frustrated with someone, betrayed, or stuck in a loop of complaining.
2. Write down exactly how you showed up in that situation.
3. Identify where you could have set a boundary, spoken up, pivoted earlier, or made a firmer decision.

January 27th

Commit to Consistent Reflection

A masculine man understands that unchecked momentum can be just as dangerous as stagnation. You don't operate mindlessly, mistaking busyness for progress. Instead, you carve out time to review your performance with brutal honesty and focused intent. This discipline of consistent reflection keeps you aligned with your mission and ensures you're not drifting, coasting, or falling into unconscious patterns. Reflection is strategic recalibration.

The masculine man doesn't just hope things will improve; he inspects the process, audits his character, and makes real-time adjustments to stay on target. Learning these skills, you evolve faster than the man who waits for life to teach him the same lesson twice.

Reflection builds pattern recognition. It reveals where energy leaks are hiding, where hesitation has stolen opportunities, and where pride might have clouded judgment. It also highlights progress, those small, decisive wins —the milestones that stack up to build your confidence. It reminds you of how far you've come, what you're building, and why it all matters.

Action:

1. Tonight, sit in silence for five minutes before sleep. Open a notebook and write three lines:

2. One thing you did well today that aligned with your purpose.

3. One decision or moment you could have handled better.

4. One adjustment you'll make tomorrow is to lead with more clarity and conviction.

January 28th

Strengthen Mental Toughness

A masculine man knows that actual toughness isn't loud, reactive, or aggressive; it's silent, grounded, and built from radical ownership. You don't crumble when life punches you hard in the face; you don't outsource blame or collapse under pressure. You step into it. Mental toughness is taking full responsibility for everything in your world: your actions, thoughts, attitude, and the outcomes that result from them. Every time you own your mistakes, instead of deflecting, you condition your mind to stay composed under pressure.

Mental strength isn't something you're born with; it's trained, rep after rep, like building muscle in the gym. When most men crack under pressure, the masculine man breathes deeper, thinks clearly, and responds with precision. You learn to reinterpret struggle as a signal, and where others see problems, you see solutions and a new training ground.

Over time, this mindset becomes your default. Pressure no longer rattles you or has any weight; it sharpens you. Adversity doesn't knock you off course; it clarifies the mission. This thought process reprograms the brain to eliminate the victim mindset and take full command of your life. That's the strength of mental toughness: controlling your breath, controlling your mind, and you control your world.

Action:

1. Pick one area of your life where you've been blaming someone or something else: money, time, a relationship, or circumstance.

2. Write down three ways you can take direct responsibility for improving it today.

3. Take one action, no matter how small, that proves to yourself you're in control.

January 29th

Take Immediate Action

For the masculine man on a path of purpose, accountability isn't just about acknowledging fault; it's about swift, decisive correction. Owning your mistake without taking action is just a confession. What separates the man who evolves from the man who repeats patterns is your ability to move with urgency the moment you see where you slipped. Masculine accountability means you don't wallow in guilt, spiral in self-criticism, or wait for the perfect time to make things right. You move now. You act because your word to yourself and others carries weight, and every second you delay is a crack in your integrity.

When you train yourself to take immediate action after a mistake, whether it's fixing a misstep, having a difficult conversation, or simply showing up with more intensity, you build a reputation that others can count on and, more importantly, a solid self-image—this kind of responsiveness compounds into an unstoppable momentum. Over time, you stop fearing failure because you know you'll always correct yourself fast. You don't stall. You don't hide. You recalibrate and get back in the game sharper than before.

This habit is vital for your purpose because a man who delays action delays impact. Your mission doesn't wait. Every time you act immediately, you reinforce that your path is non-negotiable.

Action:

1. Identify one mistake, broken commitment, or avoided responsibility you've been sitting on, something you've blamed, excused, or just ignored.
2. Write it down clearly, no sugar coating.
3. Take one bold, clear step to correct it today, not tomorrow, not next week. Whether it's sending that message, fixing that error, or showing up where you've been absent, move now.

January 30th

Create Enduring Legacy

Legacy is the ultimate scoreboard for the masculine man, not of status but of substance. It's not just what you did while you were alive but what remains standing after you're gone. A man of purpose doesn't build his life for applause or validation. He understands that true power isn't in temporary wins but in values passed down, lives impacted, and systems left behind that others rise through. Your legacy isn't a statue or a trophy; it's who you became when no one was watching and what others become because you existed.

To build a legacy, a masculine man must first lead himself with ruthless accountability and relentless intention. Every habit, every action, every word becomes part of the blueprint that others will follow or ignore. That's why you hold yourself to a higher standard when no one's looking. When your purpose aligns with your legacy, shortcuts no longer interest you.

A masculine legacy is not about creating dependency; it's about awakening strength in others and being carved in behaviour, cemented in impact, and passed on through experience. The only way to write that legacy is to live your purpose as if it matters and to live each mission as if it's bigger than you.

January 31st

The Indestructible Foundation of the Masculine Man

Everything begins and ends with purpose and accountability, which are the steel framework of masculine development. This unshakable bedrock holds your vision, your identity, and your impact in place when all your strength is needed. Trends, distractions, and the opinions of weaker men easily sway a man without purpose. A man grounded in purpose becomes immovable. He no longer chases, he attracts, and he builds.

Accountability is what sharpens that purpose into action. It's the mechanism that transforms good intentions into real-world results. Every time you take ownership of your emotions, your failures, and your outcomes, you reclaim wasted energy. You stop being reactive and start being strategic. You correct the course quickly, refine it, and recalibrate daily. In doing so, you become the kind of man others respect without needing to be loud about it because your life speaks louder than your words ever could.

Your purpose gives you direction. Accountability keeps you on track. Strip away illusions, silence doubt, and form a code of conduct that doesn't break when life gets hard. Build consistency and confidence and build your legacy. When a masculine man is locked into purpose and powered by accountability, you become a force that can't be manipulated, distracted, or stopped. You are self-led. Mission-driven and respected. Everything else stacks up on top of it.

FEBRUARY

Breath & Nervous System

Regulate your breath, dominate your emotions, and stay lethal under pressure.

Your breath is the remote control to your entire system, and most men never learn how to use it. You're here to lead, to dominate, to stay clear while others fold under chaos. This section trains the system behind your strength: your breath and nervous system. Control this, and you control the pace, the power, and the pressure of every room you walk into.

A masculine man doesn't panic; you breathe, adapt, and recalibrate. You don't react; you read, adjust, and strike with precision. When your internal world is steady, nothing external can disrupt you. That's what this month is about: building a full-spectrum command over your state, your energy, and your presence under pressure.

Stress won't be something you avoid; it'll be something you harness. Emotions won't control your behaviour; they will amplify your clarity. Breath won't just keep you alive; it will become your edge, your grounding, your new trigger for complete nervous system control.

This month isn't about calming down; it's about powering up more efficiently. You'll train your body to respond like a weapon in the chaos.

"Master your breath, and the world will
no longer control your state."

February 1st

Own Your Breath, Own the Day

Every masculine man's day should begin with a deliberate moment of ownership, and your breath is the gateway to that. Breath is power; it's your direct line to your nervous system, your emotions, and your energy. When you master it, you become unshakable, no matter what chaos the world throws at you.

Start every morning by sitting quietly with yourself, with your feet grounded and your eyes closed. Begin with deep, conscious breaths, not rushed, no distractions. Let each inhale fill you from the bottom up, expanding your diaphragm, then your chest, until your ribcage opens like an armour. Hold for two beats. Then exhale slowly until all the air is out, relaxing your face with every exhale, allowing your whole being to relax and become calm in both mind and body.

Use practices like One Breath Meditation (OBM) as your method. This simple act anchors you in the present, resets your stress levels, and creates a state of natural flow that sets the tone and pace of your breath for the entire day.

When you own your breath, you own your state of being, and that's the first step to owning your masculinity.

February 2nd

Develop Inner Control

Breath mastery is the cornerstone of inner control, a non-negotiable trait for any man who wants to lead himself and others. When you consciously direct your breath, you take the steering wheel of your nervous system. Instead of reacting to chaos, you respond with presence and intention.

Breathwork helps you reconnect with your natural breathing rhythm, enhances your oxygen capacity without force, and teaches you how to breathe in harmony with a calm and controlled physical, mental, and emotional response.

True masculinity demands emotional authority and the ability to face challenges without getting hijacked by stress or fear. Breath mastery is your direct path to that level of self-command. Practice daily and watch as your reactions shift from impulsive to intentional, from scattered to centred and build unshakeable composure in any situation.

Action:

1. 1 minute / nine breaths.
2. Close your eyes.
   > Begin to breathe calmly with nothing forced.

› When you breathe in, your breath draws in down through your nose, inflating your belly, then allow it to turn around and flow unforced through your mouth.

› Your chest or shoulders shouldn't be rising, and only with minimal movement.

› Breathe in through your nose, inflating your belly, then it turns around and flows unforced through your mouth.

› Breathe in through your nose, inflating your belly, and allow the air to flow out through your mouth.

› Think about the air as it travels through your nose all the way down, fills your belly, turns around and is gently released through your mouth as your belly deflates.

February 3rd

Connect to Your Nervous System

Breath isn't just air; it's the bridge to your body's hidden signals. Every man needs to develop an intuitive relationship with their stress response, recognising exactly when they're tense, tired, or overdriven, and taking action.

Breath Connection Reprocessing (BCR) is a forward-focused recalibration technique within the OBM Method. It captures moments of calm, clarity, and joy in real time, anchoring them in the subconscious through breath. These moments become the new triggers for your nervous system, training it to default you into peace, not panic.

BCR is not about revisiting the past; it's about rewriting your future body code.

It replaces old survival triggers with signals of power, presence, and peace.

This practice builds awareness, and awareness is power. A man who understands the inner workings of the body can act with precision and control. You don't let tension hijack your mind. You don't let fatigue make you sloppy. You stay sharp, decisive, and entirely in command.

This daily habit will train you to stay alert, aware, and always one step ahead of your stress.

Action:

1. Use a conscious breath to fully enter the present moment and feel safe, grounded, and aware.

2. Capture the State:

   As calm or joy rises (post-training, in nature, after connection, after a fantastic meal), continue breathing rhythmically to capture that moment and imprint that feeling.

   1 breath.

3. › Connect with one breath. Inhale deeply with intent, through your nose, to inflate your belly.

4. › Hold for two beats.

   › And release gently through your mouth with nothing forced.

   Anchor It:

   40 seconds / three breaths.

   › Calm your breathing with long, drawn-out breaths, focusing on seamless transitions from inhale to exhale, calming your face on every exhale.

   › Focus only on your breath and how smooth you can make it. While holding that elevated state, this locks it into your system. Repeat Often.

February 4th

Build Calm in Chaos

Masculinity cultivates in tests and challenges, and when the pressure builds, most men break. The masculine man doesn't get rattled; you remain calm, present, and in control, even when everything around you is falling apart.

That's where breath control comes in. When you own your breath, you cultivate a stable, regulated nervous system that resists panic. Each inhale is a reminder that you're in charge of your state, and each exhale releases tension and fear.

When chaos strikes, whether it's in a high-pressure meeting, a personal crisis, or a high-risk physical challenge, your breath becomes your anchor. You remain steady while others crumble. You lead, not react.

February 5th

Regulate Stress with Breath

When stress hits, most men react by tightening their shoulders, clenching their jaw, and taking short, shallow breaths, which triggers their nervous system into a state of fight-or-flight, making them react impulsively instead of responding from a place of strength.

You were born with a natural breathing rhythm that's slow, deep, and nasal-driven. Inhale through the nose, exhale through the mouth. That's because nasal breathing naturally filters and humidifies the air, triggers the diaphragm to engage, and releases nitric oxide, which improves oxygen delivery and blood flow. Holding the breath for two beats after an intentional inhale creates a slight build-up of carbon dioxide, which trains your body to tolerate stress and stay calm under pressure.

When you slow your exhale, you activate the parasympathetic nervous system, the body's natural brake pedal, telling your body, "You're safe. You can relax. You can think clearly." is crucial for a masculine man: composure and self-control separate leaders from those who react.

Action:

1. Inhale slowly through your nose for four counts
2. Hold for two counts
3. Exhale slowly through your mouth for a count of six.
4. Relax your face on every exhale.
5. Repeat this cycle five times in the morning and again at night.
6. Notice how you feel after each session.
7. Don't wait for stressful moments; practice to retrain your new, natural breathing rhythm.

February 6th

Study the Invisible

A high-level, masculine man knows that life isn't just what you can see. The invisible world isn't about fantasy or woo-woo mysticism; it's about sharpening your perception to understand cause beyond effect, a pattern beneath the surface, and the energy behind words. It's about developing depth, not falling into blind compliance or shallow thinking.

Most men operate like sheep because they only react to what they can touch or prove. The masculine edge is learning how to sit with what doesn't make immediate sense, how to observe without pushing back, and how to remain still in uncertainty without defaulting to anger, sarcasm, or arrogance.

The man who studies energy, rhythm, human behaviour, nonverbal cues, breath, tone, and intention; that man has range. You have a psychological advantage. You're not surprised by people or situations. You read them. You anticipate better. You respond rather than react. If you can't interpret what you can't see, you'll forever be at the mercy of people who can.

Action:

1. Observe without judgment. Spend 10 minutes in silence daily. No music, no screens. Watch your thoughts. Watch your body. What's agitated? What's calm? Start listening to your system like a radar, not a machine.

2. Track patterns. Notice when certain things keep happening: frustrations, delays, wins. Don't just write it off. Write it down. See the connections.

3. Read energy. Next time you walk into a room or meet someone, feel before you speak. Feel their tension. What's their breath doing? Match your presence to the moment and lead it.

February 7th

Rebuild Sensory Awareness & Overcome Early Disconnection

From birth until about age five, your senses are your primary way of engaging with the world, pure, raw, and alive. You learn by touch, sound, smell, and movement. As you grow, society teaches you to suppress these instincts. School, rules, and social expectations tell you to sit still, quiet your body, and focus on thinking over feeling. This conditioning disconnects you from your internal sensors, your body's way of signalling stress, safety, energy, and flow.

This loss dulls your edge as a masculine man because real power and presence come from full sensory integration, the ability to accurately read your environment and your body and respond in real time. Without it, you're reactive, disconnected, and easily overwhelmed.

You move in flow with the world, not against it. When your senses are sharp and your breath controlled, you hold authority over your internal state. Stress no longer hijacks you. You lead with presence and a confidence that is authentic and strong within.

Rebuilding this connection is foundational for true masculinity. It's about staying grounded in chaos, tapping into flow, and leading yourself and others without hesitation.

This intentional sensory practice recalibrates your nervous system, shifting it from a reactive to a responsive state. You move from being overwhelmed by your environment to mastering it, calm, focused, and powerful.

Action:
Each day, spend 10 minutes fully immersed in your environment, whether in nature or an urban setting.

1. Find a tree, a beach, or a busy street. Close your eyes briefly.
2. See the subtle movements, leaves fluttering, waves rolling, and people flowing.
3. Feel the breeze or the temperature on your skin.
4. Listen carefully to every sound around you: birds, wind, footsteps, engines.
5. Inhale deeply through your nose for 4 seconds, hold your breath for two beats, then exhale slowly through your mouth for 6 seconds. Let your breath sync with the rhythm of what you observe, like matching the pulse of the waves or the sway of the branches.
6. Notice how your body feels: tense, relaxed, energised, tired. Don't judge, observe.

February 8th

Reset After Challenges

Every masculine man faces pressure points: arguments, setbacks, and big decisions. When stress spikes, your body goes into fight-or-flight: tense, scattered, and reactive. Your breath is your reset button. Use controlled breathing to calm your nervous system fast and switch from survival mode to a focused presence.

Masculine mastery is about controlled power, not constant aggression. Reset fast. Lead yourself first.

Action:

1. Pause.
2. Inhale through your nose (4 counts), hold (2 counts), exhale slowly through your mouth (6 counts).
3. Repeat 3–5 times.
4. Feel tension melt.
5. Ask yourself: "What's my best next move?"
6. Act with confidence.

February 9th

Ground Yourself in the Present

Grounding means anchoring your mind and body in the present moment, connecting physically and energetically to the Earth and the world around you.

Why Grounding Matters:

- Science-backed benefits: Barefoot contact with the Earth's surface (earthing) allows the body to absorb free electrons, reducing inflammation, lowering cortisol, and balancing the autonomic nervous system.

- Vibrational alignment: The Earth's natural frequency (Schumann resonance, 7.83 Hz) aligns with your brain's alpha waves, promoting calm focus, essential for masculine leadership.

- Emotional steadiness: Grounding shifts you from fight-or-flight to calm control, making you a man who responds, not reacts.

- Relationship strength: A grounded man is present and reliable, building trust and deeper bonds with others.

When you combine intentional breathing with physical movement, such as walking barefoot, training mindfully, or simply standing still, you align your body's energy with the

Earth's natural rhythm, thereby building stamina, confidence, and emotional resilience.

Grounding isn't just about your body; it's about your mindset. It's knowing you're part of something larger, a connected living system. It's where your authentic masculine power lives: unshakeable, focused, and present.

Grounding is the foundation that transforms thoughts into action, stress into resilience, and isolation into connection. That's how you become the man who commands respect.

Action:

- Practice intentional breathing outdoors, preferably barefoot.
- Feel the Earth beneath you, with its textures, temperature, and support.
- Integrate this feeling into your training, conversations, and daily life.

February 10th

Emotional Resilience

Promoting emotional resilience through sensory-cognitive integration and breathwork is the key to handling life's emotional curveballs without losing your composure. When stress or anger hits, your breath is the first line of defence, a bridge between your rational mind and your reactive instincts.

By staying tuned in to your environment, every sound, sight, and sensation, you're training yourself to remain calm, even when emotions run hot. Breath acts as the stabiliser, keeping your nervous system grounded and preventing triggers from hijacking your decisions, moving from emotional reactivity to emotional mastery. Instead of being a man who explodes or shuts down, you become the man who stands steady in the storm, making decisions based on purpose rather than emotion.

When you consistently integrate your senses with breath, you're not just surviving; you're building a mental fortress. You're forging the kind of composure that earns respect and inspires trust.

Action:

1. When you feel an emotional trigger, whether it's anger, fear, or stress, pause.
2. Take a deep breath in, paying attention to how the environment is affecting you.
3. Hold for a moment, then exhale slowly. Feel your body relax and your mind calm.
4. Feel the ground beneath your feet.
5. Choose your response, not your reaction. That's where emotional resilience lives.

February 11th

Triggers connect to the nervous system.

Your body and mind store every significant experience, especially emotional ones, in both your brain and your body. When you encounter a situation that even vaguely resembles a past threat or intense moment (such as conflict, disappointment, or shame), your body remembers the feeling first before your thinking mind has a chance to catch up.

That feeling of tightness in your chest, heat in your face, and tension in your shoulders is your nervous system's way of bracing for impact. Your breath follows suit: it quickens, shortens, or even stops. Your subconscious and physical memory at work, replaying the same breath-and-body response you had the first time you felt that way.

It's a survival mechanism, but it also locks you into an old story. Without awareness, you react not based on the current situation but on a looped recording of your past experiences.

By practising a breath connection regularly, you train your nervous system to respond to stressors with strength, clarity, and choice. You effectively rewrite the emotional script. That's where a masculine man steps into mastery, owning your triggers, recalibrating your response, and building a new level of self-trust and power that cannot be shaken.

Here's the transformation:

1. Intentional breath practice interrupts that automatic reaction. When you breathe deeply and intentionally, you shift from your sympathetic (fight-or-flight) nervous system to your parasympathetic (rest-and-digest) state, sending a powerful signal to your brain that you are safe and can choose how to respond.

2. Sensory-cognitive integration grounds you in the present. By paying close attention to your surroundings, sounds, textures, temperatures, and even the feel of your breath, you teach your nervous system to recalibrate from past threats to present reality.

3. Body scanning helps you identify where you hold tension or emotional residue from past experiences.

4. Self-awareness, which involves consciously noticing your triggers in the moment, allows you to catch them before they take over.

5. Movement, whether it's a walk, stretching, or a powerful physical reset, forms a new pattern, allowing your body to choose a new response instead of defaulting to the old one.

Breath, Triggers, and Altered States

There's a level of self-command that you cannot access through logic or mindset hacks alone. It must be earned, not by avoiding your triggers but by stepping into them fully, on your terms. That's where deep fire breathwork comes in, not the soft, meditative kind, but the raw, unapologetic, nervous-system-resetting kind. Think Wim Hof, Somatic and Shamanic, for pattern disruption, designed to reveal what lies beneath the surface.

Top-tier masculine men don't avoid pressure. They create it intentionally. Controlled breathwork in altered states pushes your nervous system to its edge; it activates suppressed emotions, trauma, hidden fears, and old programming. Instead of running, you sit in it. Eyes closed; body engaged. You let the chaos come up, rage, shame, grief, and then you own it without pushback or judgment.

You're not here to be a polished, surface-level "leader." You're here to discover your full potential and harness it. It's about wiring your nervous system to handle pressure, triggers, pain, and power without folding. You become the man who can walk into war calmly because he's already fought the battle within.

Benefits:

- High-level clarity under emotional chaos
- Instant access to the regulation after activation
- Emotional release that creates space for sharper decision-making
- Inner trust that you've faced your dark and didn't blink
- Presence and depth that no man or woman can ignore

It separates the men who think they're in control from the men who are.

Action:

1. Block 30–45 minutes alone.
2. Lay flat.
3. Use a powerful breath sequence: 30–40 connected breaths (inhale fully through the nose, passive exhale through the mouth), then hold your breath on the exhale for as long as possible. Repeat for 3–4 rounds.
4. Let your body respond to emotions, heat, and movement. Don't resist it. Sit in it. Then finish with 3 minutes of deep, nasal breathing to calm your system and integrate.
5. Write down what came up and your next layer to work on.

Command Your Breath, Command Your Power

Controlled breathing isn't just a wellness tactic; it's a foundational weapon for masculine performance, presence, and power. A masculine man who masters his breath is a man who governs his physical, mental, and emotional state. When you breathe deeply through the nose, drawing oxygen into your diaphragm, and exhale slowly and fully through your mouth, you are doing more than just calming your nervous system. You are fuelling every organ, every muscle, and every neuron with the life force it needs to perform at its peak. This breath control becomes a hidden edge, providing more stamina in training, greater clarity in chaos, and faster recovery under stress.

Whether you're under the weight of a barbell, in the heat of a boardroom decision, or standing grounded during emotional conflict, your ability to regulate your breath dictates whether you stay composed or collapse. Shallow, erratic breathing leads to anxiety, brain fog, and early fatigue; it leaks energy. Trained, intentional breathwork locks you into the present moment, recharges your body in real time, and extends your capacity far beyond the average man. Over time, your baseline of energy rises, your patience deepens, and you transcend resilience automatically.

Every elite warrior, athlete, and leader understands this: the man who controls their breath controls their environment. It is the bridge between your internal world and your external performance. Integrate breathwork daily, and you will not just feel stronger; you will be stronger for longer and more lethal in every domain.

Align Your Breath with Movement

Breath isn't just background noise during movement; it's the ignition switch of your physical power. For the masculine man, aligning breath with movement is the practice that bridges brute strength with refined control. When your breath and body are in sync, you eliminate wasted motion, reduce mental clutter, and enter a flow state where effort becomes efficient precision. Flow state is not limited to elite athletes or martial artists; it is a foundational skill that upgrades every physical action you take, from lifting weights to running, climbing, or even walking into a room with presence.

Physiologically, your breath governs oxygen delivery, heart rate, nervous system regulation, and muscular endurance. When you inhale deeply through the nose before initiating movement, you preload the system with fuel. When you exhale fully through the mouth during execution, you release tension and activate core control. Breath becomes a metronome that sets the tempo of your effort, ensuring you don't gas out prematurely or operate in chaotic bursts. It anchors you in the present, making your body an extension of your mind. You start to move with precision rather than force and fluidity rather than friction.

Masculine mastery is not about grinding aimlessly. It's about control. It refines your capacity to make each rep, step, or strike count without wasting energy.

Action for Today:

1. During your next training session or physical task, consciously link every movement to your breath.

2. Inhale through your nose during preparation (e.g., lowering in a squat, drawing a punch back), and exhale sharply and fully through your mouth during execution (e.g., driving up, throwing the strike).

3. Stay focused on the rhythm, every breath, every rep. When your breath starts to stray, your awareness has drifted. Bring it back.

4. Repeat until the rhythm becomes automatic. Make this standard not optional.

February 15th

Use Breath to Focus

A masculine man doesn't allow his mind to scatter before stepping into battle, whether it's a high-stakes conversation, a critical workout, or a business decision. You command your state with precision, and the first tool you reach for is your breath. Before action, don't rush in reactively; centre yourself. A deliberate breath is not weakness or a pause; it's the power of choosing your mental state before the world decides it for you. When you inhale deeply through your nose, hold with control, and exhale slowly through your mouth, you're not just oxygenating your system; you're also commanding your nervous system to relax.

That breath disrupts internal chaos, breaks emotional loops, and refocuses your attention on the mission at hand. It's the reset that separates amateurs from operators. Distractions fade. Doubt dissolves. You become fully present. In that presence, the masculine man becomes lethal, decisive, calm, and effective, making your breath a weapon: one that keeps your head clear when others spiral and your path direct when others drift.

Action:

1. Before your next key task, conversation, or training session, take a moment to reflect.

2. Close your eyes. Take one deep breath in through your nose for four seconds.

3. Hold for two.

4. Exhale through your mouth for six seconds. Feel your mind sharpen. Your heartbeat is slow. Your body aligns.

5. Step forward on the exhale with absolute intent. Repeat as often as needed.

February 16th

Confidence Is Essential for the Masculine Man

Confidence isn't just a personality trait; it's a vital pillar of masculinity. Without it, a man is unstable, reactive, and easily thrown off course by challenge, rejection, or uncertainty. True confidence, the kind that commands respect and steadies entire rooms, doesn't come from ego or applause. A masculine man develops it by mastering the one realm he always controls: Your internal state. Breath and nervous system control are not soft skills; they're strategic weapons. When you can slow your breath under pressure and shift your nervous system out of panic and into a state of power, you prove to yourself that you can lead, decide, and act without being emotionally hijacked. That's absolute confidence earned through physiological command, not performative bluster.

When others break under stress, you remain grounded. When situations spiral out of control, you become the axis of stability. You know your state is your responsibility. Controlled breath shifts you from reaction to strategy, from fear to direction.

With this as your foundation, you become the one who sets the tone. People follow that kind of man because your calm is powerful and embodied. Your confidence doesn't shout; it resonates. That's the edge. Not just feeling strong but being strong mentally, emotionally, and energetically. Confidence, grounded in breath and presence, is the masculine man's signature. It's not optional. It's essential.

February 17th

Deepen Relationships

A masculine man doesn't just dominate his goals; he brings strength and presence into every connection he builds, especially with his partner. When you master your breath, you master your state, and when you master your state, you become the grounded presence others trust, especially the woman in your life.

Women don't want chaos. They don't want a man who explodes under pressure, shuts down emotionally, or transmits stress into every interaction. They want a man who feels everything and can regulate their nervous system through deliberate breathing and moment-to-moment awareness, showing her that you can hold her emotions without collapsing into your own. That's what makes a man magnetic: not just strength but calm command.

Breath grounds you in the now. It rewires old triggers, stops emotional reactivity before it escalates, and helps you stay composed when conversations get tough. When your nervous system remains calm, your words are clear, your energy is stable, and your touch is gentle and safe. That stability creates space for vulnerability, passion, and intimacy. It's not just softness; it's power under control, which makes deep, lasting relationships. Not performance. No promises, but the man who shows up clear, calm, and fully present, day in, day out.

Action:

1. Breath gives you access to emotional leadership, not emotional suppression.

2. Sensory awareness makes you more attuned to your partner's needs before words are spoken.

3. Nervous system control ensures your presence is safe, reliable, and trusted, especially during times of conflict.

4. Ownership of your state builds unshakable respect because she knows you don't shift with the wind.

February 18th

Breathe Before You Choose

For the masculine man, breath is more than a stress-relief tool; it's a means of grounding oneself in truth, presence, and discernment in high-stakes moments, especially in love. Calm, intentional breathing sharpens your self-awareness, allowing you to avoid chasing validation or reacting impulsively.

When you breathe with control, you are no longer at the mercy of chemistry alone. You start to feel the alignment, not just the attraction. You begin to recognise what's real and what's a projection of past wounds or unmet needs. Breath grounds you into the clarity to see red flags before they become regrets. You trust yourself more deeply, and that self-trust becomes the compass for choosing the right partner, not based on fear of being alone, but from a solid place of grounded wholeness.

When it comes to taking risks, starting the conversation, making the approach, and opening your heart, your breath becomes the switch that calms the nervous system and channels confidence. You're not chasing approval. You're offering presence. Women immediately sense that a man who is in command of his breath carries an energy that says, "I'm not here to impress; I'm here because I know who I am."

February 19th

Sharpening the Senses

Sight isn't just about what's in front of you. It's about how you perceive, assess, and respond to the world around you, and that makes it one of the most powerful tools in the masculine man's arsenal. A man who sees more widely and more deeply holds a distinct edge over the one who merely looks. Your eyes are a direct extension of your brain and nervous system. What you see, how you interpret it, motion, depth, and energy all directly impact your decisions, emotions, and sense of control.

In today's overstimulated world, many men live in a state of visual tunnel vision, locked into screens, narrowly focused, and reactive. This constriction increases stress, reduces situational awareness, and shrinks confidence. When you retrain your eyes to expand, to scan wider than your periphery, to reach further than the horizon, you shift from reactivity to command. You begin to see not just objects but patterns. You read people's energy. You notice subtle opportunities others miss. You lead because you see it first.

Practising intentional sight isn't just tactical; it's spiritual. It demands curiosity, stillness, and a sense of presence. When you pair sight work with grounded breathing, you regulate your nervous system while heightening your perception. Your gaze becomes steady, not jumpy. You take in a room with calm dominance, not rushed anxiety. This practice enables you to pause and respond instead of reacting, whether in a high-stakes conversation, a conflict, or a leadership moment.

Action:

1. Peripheral Vision Expansion:

    Stand barefoot or with feet firmly grounded.

    Take a slow, deep inhale through your nose, expanding your belly. Hold for a second, then exhale slowly through your mouth.

    While breathing, soften your gaze and widen your awareness of the edges of your vision. Notice colours, movement, and shadows to reduce stress and increase environmental awareness.

2. Near-Far Focus Drills:

    While grounded, breathe deeply and choose an object close to you. Focus on the details, texture, edges, and shadows.

    Exhale slowly, then shift your focus to something far away (tree, horizon).

    Repeat, letting your breath set the rhythm, training your eyes and nervous system to adapt and stay present under pressure.

3. 360-Degree awareness:

    Ground yourself in the environment by planting your feet and maintaining a tall posture.

    With each breath, let your eyes explore up, down, and side to side, noticing details without judgment.

    This exercise trains your brain to scan for threats and opportunities, building confidence and calm.

February 20th

Command Through Listening

A masculine man isn't just defined by what he says or does but by how deeply he listens, cultivating an alert stillness and an awareness that draws power from what most men ignore. In a world flooded with surface-level noise, opinions, pressure, and false urgency, a grounded man filters through the chaos by tuning into the only signals that matter.

To listen is to trust that your instincts are built from truth, earned through pain, and refined by presence. When you master the ability to synchronise your breath and awareness with your environment, you don't just hear the world; you own your place in it.

Action:

- Start with Breath: Pause. Inhale deeply through your nose, hold briefly, and exhale longer than you inhale. Let your breath around you.
- Scan Your Body: Release any tension or tightness; these are signals from within.
- Observe Your Surroundings: Feel the ground, listen to the environment, and engage your senses.

- Listen to the Whisper: The loud voices are demands; the quiet voice is your truth. Trust the calm, intuitive insights.
- Take Action: Once you've listened, move. Masculinity requires decisive action, not just reflection.

February 21st

Transcend Resilience

Resilience is survival. You can take a hit, fall, and get back up. That's respectable, but it's not the masculine way. The masculine man doesn't train to bounce back; you now train to rise above.

In the modern world, resilience has become a safe word. A soft landing. Resilience says, "You've been through pain, and you're still standing." Masculine transcendence says, "I turned that pain into fuel, and now I stand taller than ever."

True masculine strength isn't about returning to baseline. It's about permanently upgrading it. You don't just recover. You recalibrate. You use the hardship, the pressure, and the setback not to repair the old version of yourself but to take you to the next level.

When you transcend resilience, your nervous system becomes a weapon, not just regulated but optimised. Your breath is not just calming; it's commanding. Your focus isn't scattered; it's locked in. You're not waiting for the hits so you can prove you'll recover. You're moving first, with clarity and force. You no longer bounce back. You break through.

What Happens When the Masculine Man Transcends Resilience

When a masculine man transcends resilience, your identity stops being rooted in the past and is now redefined by who you become every time you face another test. Where most shrink back into comfort, you step forward with calculated action, knowing life flows for the man who keeps moving forward with purpose.

In business, you lead without hesitation. While others drown in indecision, you operate from clarity and calm. Chaos doesn't faze you. You make bold moves not out of ego but from earned confidence. You become the man others look to, not for hype, but for direction, for solutions, for grounded strength when the pressure hits hardest. Your reputation becomes bulletproof because you deliver consistently without needing praise.

In your physical pursuit, you stop counting reps and start measuring your capacity for evolution. Training isn't about fatigue or grinding anymore; it's about command. Your breath becomes your weapon. Your focus becomes surgical. Your body is tuned, adapted, and battle tested. You build yourself to be ready every day in every situation.

In your relationship, you don't just show up; you lead with depth. Emotional spikes don't break you; they sharpen your emotional intelligence, enabling you to hold space like a warrior monk: calm in chaos, fierce in loyalty, and present with purpose.

Every day, through breath, clarity, and decisive action, you reclaim more of yourself and take life to places that others dare not even imagine.

February 23rd

Command Dominance and Respect, Without Raising Your Voice

A truly masculine man doesn't need to yell, threaten, or posture to dominate. His presence does the work long before he speaks. When you've mastered your breath, sharpened your senses, and taken ruthless ownership of every choice and outcome, you radiate something rare: an unshakable presence. It's a calm intensity that fills the space. Not from ego. Not from force. From a deep internal command that others instinctively recognise and respect.

Through doing the hard work in silence while others perform for applause. You move with intention, grounded in your body, locked in your vision, and that's why people trust you. They know you won't collapse under pressure, react emotionally, or break down when life gets hard.

You lead yourself so powerfully that others naturally align with your direction. You've built a centre of gravity so intense it pulls people in. When you enter a room, your energy says everything without needing to prove anything.

Action:

1. Start with your posture.
2. Ground your feet into the ground.
3. Relax your jaw. Shoulders back.
4. Breathe slowly and deeply in through your nose, out through your mouth.
5. When you speak, do so on the out-breath, with weight, calm, measured, and deliberate.
6. Let silence follow your words when needed.
7. Walk into every room like the outcome already bends in your favour.

The Irresistible Aura of Deep Masculine Man

A masculine man who embodies deep mastery doesn't need noise, bravado, or dominance. His aura does the work before he says a word.

Women feel this instantly, not through logic, but through biology. Their nervous system picks it up like a radar. A man with high heart rate variability, calm breath patterns, and a stable nervous system sends a signal of safety, strength, and sexual polarity. That's what draws women in: the emotional steadiness, the energetic charge of a man who doesn't need anything but chooses with precision. He becomes magnetic, not through pursuit, but through presence.

Other men feel it, too, but differently. They don't always know what it is; they sense tension around you because your grounded energy becomes a mirror. Their untrained, reactive selves are exposed. You don't need to say a word, and yet their insecurities rise to the surface. That discomfort is not intimidation; it's showing them what they haven't yet faced within.

Ask: "Do I need to take control, or can I be the control?" Watch how people respond

Here's why it works:

1. HRV (Heart Rate Variability) + Vagal Tone: A calm nervous system with high HRV signals strength and leadership. It shows a man in control, not ruled by emotion or threat, which puts others, especially women, at ease and draws them in.

2. Energetic Frequency: When you slow down your internal world, your external field expands. Vibrational physics operates at low frequencies and is characterised by chaos, whereas high frequencies are more controlled and precise. A regulated man resonates at a frequency that soothes women and challenges men.

February 25th

Breath & Affirmation Ritual

A masculine man doesn't rely on hype, noise, or surface-level affirmations pulled from a social media post; he builds unshakable confidence from within. Your affirmations shouldn't be borrowed words; they should be grounded in real achievement, forged through your pain, failures, and victories and owned through your breath connection. When you breathe into an affirmation, it isn't wishful thinking; it's a reminder of who you already are. You don't say, "I am strong," with the hope of feeling it. You say it because you're already carrying weight most men never would. You don't whisper, "I am capable," to boost your self-esteem; you affirm what you've already proven to yourself again and again.

Before you step into any high-stakes moment — whether it's a meeting, a confrontation, a date, a challenge, or a high-risk event —pause and draw a deep, steady breath through your nose, filling your diaphragm. On the exhale, you lock eyes with the moment ahead and affirm what you know to be true—not based on hope, but on a history of your success, training your body and mind to connect action with self-belief. Over time, you don't just say these affirmations; you embody them. You become your coach and motivator. That's real power: a man who carries proof, breathes with control, and never forgets what you've already conquered.

February 26th

Close the Day with Breath

A masculine man knows that how he closes the day defines how he wakes up the next day. Ending each day with intentional breathwork is not just a ritual; it's a powerful tool for releasing tension, integrating the day's lessons, and preparing for deep, restorative sleep.

Closing the day with breath honours your connection to larger cycles: the sun's setting, the moon's rise, and Earth's 7.83 Hz Schumann Resonance. This rhythm supports deep sleep and mental clarity, ensuring you wake grounded, strong, and ready to lead. You're a man who can ground yourself in a breath at day's end and own your emotions, actions, and intentions. You lead yourself first, with no excuses and no distractions. You align your biology, mind, and spirit to be ready to dominate tomorrow's challenges with clarity and strength.

Action:

1. Set the Scene

    To Find a quiet space, dim the lights, and remove distractions.

    Sit upright in a relaxed posture.

2. Breathe Intentionally

   Or Inhale slowly through the nose for a count of 4, feeling your diaphragm expand.

   Hold gently for a count of 2, acknowledging the stillness between inhale and exhale.

   Exhale slowly through the mouth for a count of 6, feeling calm throughout your body.

3. Reflect and Integrate

   On each inhale,

   Ask yourself: "What did I learn today? What will I do differently tomorrow?"

   On each exhale,

   Let the answers flow without force and a sense of gratitude and acceptance.

4. Visualise Restoration

   Imagine your body recharging, cells rebuilding, and your nervous system recalibrating.

February 27th

Breath, Frequency & Wealth

Wealth isn't just about effort; it's about energetic alignment. The most elite masculine men don't rely on brute force alone; they move with inner stillness, breathing with intent and calibrating their nervous system to the frequency of prosperity, thereby building a grounded nervous system, mastery, cognitive clarity, and embodied authority.

Slow, deep breathing tones your vagus nerve, activates your parasympathetic system and puts you into a dominant alpha state, where you are calm, aware, and magnetically focused. Pair that with tonal frequencies like 432Hz (harmony) or 528Hz (transformation), and you shift from scattered to strategic. You stop chasing wealth and start attracting it through presence, decisiveness, and grounded energy.

That's the edge I witness in high-level men who work with me, tapping into it fast, building mental clarity, physical stamina, increasing wealth, and the kind of quiet power that turns vision into execution.

Action:

1. Put on 528Hz or 432Hz tone in your headphones.
2. Sit in stillness.

3. Breathe in through your nose for 7 seconds, hold for 2, and exhale slowly for 7.

4. Visualise your most powerful future self, already calm, clear, and wealthy.

5. Do this for 3 minutes.

6. Now execute.

February 28th

The Rare Breed

A high-level masculine man is not just confident; You are relevant, embodied, and unshakably accountable. You operate with a presence that is felt before you speak and remembered long after you leave. This level of masculinity isn't handed down or mimicked; it's earned through relentless internal work forged in solitude, pressure, and truth. You live what you teach. While others perform masculinity, you are grounded, precise, aware, and dangerous in the best possible way.

You refine your physical body without obsession, sharpen your mind without arrogance, and cultivate emotional discipline without shame. You breathe with intention, feel deeply without losing control, and integrate those sensations into deliberate, effective action. Every challenge you face becomes a test of that integration. You don't rise to the occasion; you default to your training.

Most men never reach this level because it demands too much truth. It forces them to confront every weakness, to live without excuses, without handholding and shortcuts. It's not about being better than others; it's about never settling for less than your value every day.

In a world full of distractions, weak role models, and reactive energy, you stand as the rare signal of power, direction, and grounded masculinity.

March

Style & Presence

Your presence speaks before you do. Make it say power, precision, and unshakable certainty

Before you speak, the world has already judged you. The question is, did you say 'power' or 'permission'? This section isn't about fashion. It's about presentation as domination. It's about controlling the energy you broadcast before a word ever leaves your mouth. Masculine presence is silent authority, and you're here to own it.

Your appearance, your posture, your eye contact, your scent, your stillness, every detail is a signal. Whether you like it or not, people are always listening to those signals. The masculine man doesn't try to impress. You refine. You sharpen. You eliminate anything soft, sloppy, or uncertain until even your silence has weight.

This month is about commanding space, not filling it. You'll calibrate your style to match your identity. You'll strip away anything that doesn't project strength, clarity, and intention.

You'll become the man who shifts the room by entering it without needing to posture, flex, or speak.

You're not just building a look. You're building a legacy in motion.

"Style is not what you wear; it's how you carry the man you've become."

March 1st

Dress to Command Respect

A masculine man understands that how you dress is a powerful nonverbal message about who you are. Well-fitted, tailored clothes signal to the world and yourself that you take pride in your presence. Quality over quantity is key; own fewer pieces that speak volumes.

Psychological studies consistently show that clothing affects not only how others perceive you but also how you perceive yourself, known as "enclothed cognition." Wearing well-chosen, fitted clothes triggers a boost in testosterone, confidence, and risk-taking behaviours, core masculine traits that position you as a leader, not a follower.

Action:

1. Off-the-rack is a start, but nothing commands respect like a shirt or jacket tailored to your unique build.
2. Start by going into your wardrobe and selecting one outfit (a blazer, trousers, shirt, or t-shirt) and get it tailored. Shoulders, waist, and sleeve length are essential considerations.

March 2nd

Instant Respect Starts with Presence and Precision

When you walk into a room grounded in authenticity, internal control, and tailored purpose, dressed to suit the moment, carrying the calm of a man who knows exactly who he is, the dynamic shifts. You don't need to speak first. The way you hold yourself, the way your eyes move, and how you breathe already set the tone and masculine presence.

Instant respect isn't something you demand; it's something you command by how you lead yourself. People instantly recognise a man who has done the work and who doesn't need to posture or perform. They know you are the one in the room who won't break under pressure. That speaks louder than any introduction.

When the time comes for meetings, a masculine man introduces himself with purpose. To another man, it's eye contact, a firm handshake, and your name is spoken clearly and not rushed. The handshake is an energy exchange. Not aggressive, not limp; it's the physical affirmation of your presence: steady, strong, and grounded. You're not here to dominate; you're here to connect from a place of mutual respect.

When meeting a woman, the same rule of presence applies, but the energy shifts. If it's a social setting, the introduction is warm, open, and respectful. A slight touch on the back of the hand or a nod paired with your name shows confidence without overstepping. In a professional context, your handshake remains the same: steady, intentional, brief but intense; a. A man who treats her as an equal and still holds the line of refined masculine energy gains her trust and respect.

Action:

1. Next time you enter a room, pause at the door.
2. Take one deep breath into the belly.
3. Level your posture, roll your shoulders back, and soften your facial expression.
4. Walk in with calm, directed intent.
5. Greet someone and speak your name clearly, maintaining eye contact.
6. Practice the handshake until it becomes second nature: firm, present, and respectful every time.

March 3rd

Master the Fit, Not the Flash

The real power in masculine style doesn't come from the label; it comes from the fit. You can wear a basic $50 tee and look like a force or wear a $5,000 suit and look like a lost boy drowning in fabric. The fit lies between respect and ridicule. Every piece of clothing you wear should contour your physique, not suffocate it, and not hang off it. It should shape your shoulders, define your waist, skim your arms and legs, complement the frame you've built or are building and understand your body and dress with precision.

The fit communicates intention. It says, 'I've thought about how I show up in the world.' That sends a message before you even open your mouth. Oversized hoodies, baggy pants, and sloppy collars all blur your shape and dilute your presence. A masculine man doesn't blur. You define. You sharpen. You reveal your structure in your decisions, movement, and clothing.

You're not just putting on clothes; you're framing your power. In a world full of men screaming for attention with trends and logos, the man who fits his clothes with quiet control always wins the room.

March 4th

Instant Credibility

In the first five seconds of meeting you, people decide how seriously to take you, and it happens before you even speak. Your appearance is either building trust or quietly disqualifying you. When you walk in looking sharp, structured, and intentional, people assume you are competent. They assume leadership. They think you've got your life together. That's the power of presentation.

It's not about being flashy; it's about showing control. Well-fitted clothes, clean grooming, composed posture, and deliberate movement all signal effort, awareness, and excellence. When you take the time to show up polished, it tells the world: If I care this much about myself, I'll care even more about the things I lead and protect. That creates unspoken confidence in you, especially in business, in leadership, and with women. People don't wait for you to earn credibility; they scan you for proof that you've already earned it. Show up sharp, and you fast-track trust, respect, and authority without saying a word. That's not fashion; that's strategic identity.

March 5th

Natural Confidence

When you look sharp, you feel sharp. A masculine man who understands his style and dresses with purpose sends an immediate message: You're self-assured, grounded, and in control. It's about wearing clothes that align with who you are on the inside. Your wardrobe should reflect your values, personality, and purpose, not a costume to impress others.

Authenticity is key here. When your clothes fit well, are tailored to your build, and suit the occasion, they signal that you pay attention to detail and respect yourself and those around you. This quiet confidence radiates a powerful, magnetic energy that others instantly sense. You become someone who doesn't need to announce their worth because their presence speaks for itself, and the difference between a man who chases validation and one who commands respect by simply being himself with confidence. When your clothing choices align with and express your true nature, you naturally feel more at ease in your skin. This sense of comfort and alignment between your inner self and your external presentation creates a level of confidence that's unshakable, even in the face of challenges.

Let go of insecurity and be present within yourself. Feel the energy of the room and the power you now hold within. If you feel it, add a slight smile of confidence and pride when you enter a room; people will instinctively take notice.

Action:

1. Before you walk into any room, pause for a moment.
2. Take one deep, controlled breath, inhale through the nose, and exhale slowly through the mouth.
3. Let that breath around you.
4. Then step forward with your shoulders relaxed, head held high, and eyes focused straight ahead. Let your steps be intentional, measured, and confident.
5. Let the room know you're there without a word.

March 6th

Magnetic Presence

When your energy aligns with your clothes and your vibe, it's like flipping a switch that radiates confidence and authenticity. The way you dress and groom yourself reflects your inner world: your values, your discipline, your self-respect.

People can sense when a man is at ease in his skin. It shows in the way you move, how you hold yourself, and the subtle cues that radiate from your energy. When you dress in a way that enhances rather than competes with who you are, you send a clear message: you know yourself, and you stand by it.

This magnetic presence is a powerful force. It makes people look twice, lean in, and pay attention without needing to say a word. Women can't help but notice the quiet confidence that radiates from you. Other men feel a silent challenge to step up their own game.

You don't have to force respect; it is a natural reaction because you embody it. That's why dressing with intention and authenticity is more than just a style choice; it's an extension of your masculine energy. It's how you become the man others want to follow, not because you're loud but because you're real.

March 7th

Know What Women Notice

Women notice everything, especially the details most men dismiss. The polish on your shoes, the cut of your shirt, the way your scent lingers without overpowering, the watch you wear, and whether you chose it with meaning or just convenience. To a discerning woman, none of this is accidental—these cues from the language of your masculine presence: quiet, refined, and undeniable.

Presence isn't just how you look; it's how you connect. The masculine man knows that to be truly captivating, you must be interested, not interesting, meaning asking better questions, listening without needing to impress, and creating space for her to express herself fully. Most men try too hard to be the highlight of the room, but the grounded man makes the woman feel like she is.

Your depth needs to match your stillness. Being well-travelled doesn't mean racking up passport stamps; it means you've tasted culture, experienced discomfort, eaten with locals, slept under the stars, missed flights, and found peace in chaos. It shows in how you carry on a conversation; you don't dominate it; you guide it. You allow her passions to surface while maintaining your presence. You share your own experiences in measured tones, demonstrating your ability to hold space while still maintaining a frame, which is what sets high-level, masculine men apart.

Action:

1. Start your day by taking five extra minutes to check your outfit and grooming.
2. Polish your shoes, smooth your collar, and select an intentional watch or accessory.

March 8th

Create Unshakeable Confidence

Unshakeable confidence isn't gifted. It's built through ownership of your outcomes, honest self-reflection, and the discipline to keep showing up, even when no one's watching.

A masculine man doesn't wait until he feels confident to act; you act in alignment with the man you're becoming, and confidence follows. It starts internally: owning your mistakes, learning from failure, and taking complete control of your direction. It's also expressed externally through how you present yourself to the world.

Looking sharp in well-fitting clothes isn't about vanity; it's about self-respect. When your style is intentional, when your body is toned, and your clothes fit with purpose, you send a message to yourself and everyone else that you're dialled in, not drifting. Your appearance reflects the internal standard you've set. Every piece of the puzzle matters: how you carry yourself, how you speak, how you walk into a room. That kind of presence doesn't need to beg for attention; it commands it.

Confidence becomes unshakeable when your inner discipline and outer expression are aligned. You know who you are, and you show it without saying a word. Confidence is built in motion, amplified by your appearance, reinforced by your presence, and backed by discipline.

Action:

1. Look at yourself in the mirror and ask: "Does what I'm wearing reflect the man I say I am?" If not, change it.
2. Put on something that fits right, feels strong, and enhances your posture.
3. Handle something you've been avoiding.

March 9th

Wear for the Moment, Not the Ego

Masculine style isn't about trying to stand out; it's about belonging with a sense of dominance. A man who truly owns himself doesn't dress to impress others; you dress with context, awareness, and purpose. Every environment has its own energy and unspoken rules. The gym demands movement and function. The boardroom demands authority. A dinner demands elegance. An airport demands ease with readiness. A date night? Presence and sexual polarity.

You don't just throw on clothes; you gear up for the moment. That means understanding the language of clothing in each space and translating it into a masculine presence. Not overdressed. Not underdressed and always dialled in. That's what makes people pay attention, not because you're loud, but because you look like you belong, like you've earned the right to be there, and like you might just be running the whole thing.

Most men get it wrong; they confuse ego with elegance. They try to be seen, not to lead. You're not peacocking for attention. You're showing respect for the space by being the man that space needs. Style with emotional intelligence, and it's a quiet power few men ever master.

Hold Yourself to a Higher Standard

A masculine man doesn't wait for society to hand him a blueprint for greatness; he writes his own and holds it with unwavering discipline. You don't outsource standards to trends or moods. You create them, maintain them, and ensure that every aspect of your life reflects them.

It's how you present yourself to others and how you handle yourself when no one's watching, from the condition of your shoes to the inside of your car. Whether it's a modest ride or a high-performance machine, it reflects your lifestyle. Keep it clean. Inside and out. A masculine man chooses a vehicle that fits his identity, not one that impresses others but one that speaks to who he is. If you're a car guy, then own that. Don't drive something that insults your ambition. Drive something that mirrors it.

Just like your watch, your shoes, your haircut, it's all data. People read it whether they're conscious of it or not.

When you step out of that car, your presence needs to match. Tailored clothing doesn't mean expensive; it means intentional. Sharp grooming doesn't mean vanity; it means self-respect. Posture, eye contact, and breath control aren't accessories.

They are the armour of a man who's leading himself at the highest level.

Does the man in the mirror and the world reflect the standard you claim to live by? Or are you cutting corners where you think no one would notice?

Raise the bar because you know your mission demands it. Don't carry yourself like an average man; be a high-level, masculine man.

Action:

1. Clean your car, both inside and out. No excuses. Make it reflect the same level of discipline you want in your life.
2. Audit your daily appearance. Are you dressing to express your standard, or just dressing to get through the day?
3. Create a 5-minute pre-departure ritual. Before you leave home or your car, straighten your collar, adjust your posture, and control your breath.
4. Enter every room as if you belong at the top.

March 11th

Attract Respect and Leadership

Authentic leadership isn't about position, rank, or external validation; it's the natural result of how a man commands himself. A high-level, masculine man never begs for respect or attempts to dominate through noise or intimidation. He earns it consistently, silently, and undeniably through how you show up in the moments most others would fold.

Leadership, for you, begins with absolute self-accountability. It's how you respond when things fall apart, when a plan fails, and when emotions run high. Instead of pointing fingers, you turn inward, own your role, and make necessary corrections without drama or delay. In a world where most men dodge responsibility, the man who carries it without flinching instantly becomes a stabilising force. You don't need to shout for others to hear you; your calm under pressure speaks volumes. When you make a mistake, you don't cover it with false confidence. You address it directly, learn quickly, and move forward with precision. That integrity builds trust from partners, peers, and everyone who sees the weight you're willing to carry on your own back.

You lead yourself first, through every routine, every discipline, every honest evaluation, long before you lead anyone else. Respect isn't the goal; it's the natural by-product of who you've chosen to become.

March 12th

Groom Like It's a Ritual

Grooming isn't vanity; it's self-command. A man of refinement treats his grooming like a ritual of precision. Your hair is neat or intentionally styled. Beard trimmed with clean edges or clean-shaven with purpose. Skin cared for, not neglected. Nails clipped, not chewed. Every detail sends a message, and the message is: I can take care of myself.

You're not doing this to be pretty. You're doing it because the way you present yourself reflects how seriously you take your mission. The world, especially women, pick up on it immediately. Clean men are respected. Sharp men are trusted. Polished men have a last effect, and when your grooming is on point, your confidence is present.

There's no place for the lazy or careless here. Masculine energy is sharpened through discipline, and grooming serves as a daily reset, reminding you that you are the standard. Ritual creates identity, and the world will treat you accordingly.

Action:

1. Audit your grooming from top to bottom, including hair, beard, skin, nails, and scent.

2. Choose one area you've been neglecting and upgrade it today.

3. Book that haircut.

4. Buy that skincare.

5. Sharpen your edges.

March 13th

Master the Details

Real men don't scream for attention through excess. They signal strength through restraint. That's where the details come in. Grooming is clean, not overdone. The scent is subtle but unforgettable, layered with intent, not sprayed with desperation. Materials are of high quality, not because of their logos, but because of how they feel on the body and how they move with you. Accessories are sharp, minimal, and enduring: a ring that holds meaning, a timepiece that tells a legacy, not a trend.

Masculinity lives in these small, disciplined choices. Anyone can wear something expensive. Few people know how to wear something intentionally. When you master the details, you control perception before a word is spoken. You walk into the room, and people notice, not because you're trying to stand out, but because everything about you says, I'm intentional.

Your presence becomes a language. Quiet. Refined. Unmistakable. In a world addicted to overexposure, the man who moves with calculated restraint always owns the room.

Scent Suggestions

Tom Ford – Oud Wood

- Warm, smoky, woody, elite without trying.

- Clean dominance. Sophisticated edge. Universally respected.
- Signature scent energy for quiet authority.

Creed – Aventus

- Pineapple, birch, musk, powerful and timeless.
- Smells like success and unapologetic masculinity.
- Women are magnetically drawn to it. Period.

Dior – Sauvage Elixir (Not the regular Sauvage)

- Deep lavender, spices, and woods.
- Rugged elegance with beast-mode performance.

Amouage – Interlude Man

- Dark incense, leather, amber, complex and unapologetically bold.
- A storm in a bottle. For the man who leads from the shadows and still dominates the light.

Activate The Energy Women Feel

Masculine presence doesn't chase attention; it commands energy, and women feel it instantly. It's not about being the loudest in the room or having the flashiest clothes. It's about being grounded in your body, your energy, and your intention. When a man walks like he owns the moment, not arrogantly, but with grounded certainty, you shift the room.

Women don't consciously analyse your style; they feel it. From the weight of your boots on the floor to the low hum of your voice tone to the scent that lingers after you walk past, it's all energetic. You're holding a frame that invites her to soften, to feel safe, to feel seen.

It starts with how you dress. Well-fitted clothes that frame your strength, not hide it. Textures that feel intentional. Accessories that tell a story. Scent that doesn't shout but stays in a woman's memory. When every part of you is aligned —body, style, voice, and eye contact —she doesn't just notice you. She feels drawn to you without even knowing why.

March 15th

Lower Your Voice, Sharpen Your Words

Masculine power isn't just about being seen; it's about being heard. Your voice is one of your most potent tools of influence, and how you use it reveals everything about your inner state. Speak slowly. Speak calmly. Lower your tone just slightly, not as an act, but from a place of being grounded. The masculine man doesn't rush to fill the silence. You aren't afraid of pauses. You're comfortable letting your words land.

When you speak like a man who believes his words carry weight, people lean in. Your tone is resonant, your words deliberate, and your message stripped of empty talk. No filler. No rambling. No senseless small talk. Every sentence should have a purpose. You don't need volume to dominate. You need precision in a substantial volume.

Women hear certainty and confidence in a composed tone. Men hear leadership. The world hears a man who knows exactly who he is and doesn't need to say much to prove it. When your voice matches your presence, you become the kind of man people stop to listen to, not out of obligation but because they feel they should.

March 16th

Be Physically Dialled In

Your body is your foundation. It's the first signal of discipline, self-respect, and strength long before you speak or move. A masculine man doesn't chase aesthetics for vanity. He trains to be prepared, composed, and capable. A strong frame doesn't just look powerful; it feels powerful. It grounds your energy. It stabilises your presence. It changes how people react around you.

When your physique aligns with your style, everything falls into place. Clothes fall better. Posture sharpens. Movement becomes intentional. You don't have to puff your chest or take up space; your body already holds it. Whether you're in a t-shirt or a tailored suit, your presence says: This man can handle himself and anything thrown at him.

Training your body isn't just lifting weights; it's reclaiming your edge. Cardio, strength, fighting ability, mobility, and posture all play a role. A masculine man walks like he can handle pressure, move with precision, and endure what others avoid. Women feel that quiet physical command is a primal signal of safety, protection, and leadership.

Accessorise Like a Signature, not a Sales Pitch

Accessories are not noise; they're statements. A masculine man doesn't wear jewellery to stand out. You select pieces that represent who you are—a raw stone pendant from a defining chapter. A vintage timepiece passed down or earned. A minimal ring that reflects edge, discipline, or intention. These aren't just fashion choices; they're part of your identity.

Every item you wear should mean something. It should speak without volume. You're not trying to dazzle; you're building presence through significance. That presence builds intrigue. People sense when your style isn't just decoration but declaration. You don't accessorise to stand out. You do it to signal that I'm proud of who I am and that every part of me is chosen with purpose.

Action:

1. Choose one accessory you already wear or one you've been thinking about and assign it meaning. If it doesn't represent something real, replace it.

2. Pick or invest in one item that speaks to who you are becoming, not who you're trying to impress.

3. From today forward, every item on your body tells your story, not a trend.

March 18th

Be Remembered, Not Just Seen

Most men get noticed for a second. The masculine man makes a lasting impact. Not because you're loud, flashy, or demanding space, but because your presence leaves a mark. The scent you wear lingers. Your eye contact is calm but surgical. Your posture is grounded. Your movements are intentional and never rushed. Everything about you feels composed, dialled in, and deliberate.

It's the difference between showing up and arriving. You don't need to dominate the room; you alter the energy in it. You speak with clarity. Pauses with weight. You wear your style as an extension of your character, not for attention, but because it's a reflection of who you are. That kind of man doesn't fade into memory. He imprints a mark of real masculine presence: You don't just pass through a room; you create a moment in it. You don't chase attention; you make others feel something they remember long after you're gone.

Action:

1. Before you leave the house, check: is what you're wearing, how you're moving, and how you're carrying yourself in alignment with the man you want to be?

2. Adjust one detail, scent, accessory, pace, or tone, and step into the room like a man not to be forgotten.

March 19th

Women Feel Both Safe and Electrified

The feminine doesn't respond to noise; she responds to energy. Nothing captivates her more than a man who can ground her chaos and ignite her desire in the same breath. That's in your grooming: sharp, clean, and intentional. It's in your wardrobe, fitted, masculine, without trying too hard. It's in the way you sit still, make eye contact, and speak with calm certainty. That presence makes her feel protected and awakened at the same time.

She's not attracted to a man who seeks to impress. She's drawn to the one who carries himself like a warrior in control. She wants to feel your strength without you having to flex. She wants to feel your direction without you controlling her. Your energy says, 'I've got this.' Your style reinforces it. Your tone delivers it. Your restraint makes her lean in further. The masculine man who gets this doesn't just look good; he feels powerful, and she feels it too, in her body, her breath, her eyes, without understanding why.

That's the secret. It's not what you wear; it's how you wear it. With purpose. With depth. With presence.

Action:

1. Before your next interaction with a woman, date, meeting, or passing moment, ask yourself: Am I grounded, clean, and composed enough to make her feel safe? Am I sharp and dialled in enough to light her up?

2. Adjust one layer: your grooming, scent, or voice tone. Then, hold the space, expressing both calm and charge.

March 20th

Show Restraint

A masculine man doesn't overshare to be understood, overreact to feel seen, or over-explain to be accepted. You move with restraint, not out of fear, but because you know the value of silence, discipline, and mystery. When you hold your words, you have your frame. When you stay calm under pressure, you show emotions that don't control you; you are driven by purpose.

In conversation, speak when it matters. Say less but make every word land. In conflict, don't flinch or escalate; stay grounded and deliberate. In decision-making, take your time to respond, not out of hesitation but because you don't operate on impulse. You own your emotions; they don't own you.

Restraint shows maturity, clarity, and control, and both men and women feel it. It creates space, tension, and respect. You don't need to prove anything. You don't need to be everywhere or say everything. When you speak less, people listen more. When you move less, people watch more closely. That's how leaders, warriors, and kings move: not to be liked but to be unforgettable.

Action:

1. In your following conversation, practice intentional restraint. Say 20% less.
2. Don't fill silences.
3. Hold eye contact.
4. Speak only what adds weight.
5. Let people feel the strength behind what you don't say.

March 21st

You Don't Need to Prove Dominance, You Embody It

True masculine dominance doesn't come from aggression, arrogance, or volume; it comes from alignment. When your outer world, including your style, grooming, and posture, reflects the inner world of your standards, discipline, and mindset, you become undeniable. There's no need to announce yourself. Your presence speaks before you do.

You're not chasing approval, trying to outperform, or projecting false confidence. You've done the inner work. You've built the discipline. Your appearance is just the exclamation point, and when that alignment is clean, people sense it instantly, in your walk, in your voice, in the way you hold space without rushing to fill it.

It's rare because most men are either polished on the outside and hollow inside or strong within but careless with how they present themselves. The man who aligns both is the man who becomes the standard without needing to say a word.

From Underwear to Overcoat, Sex Appeal is a Strategy

Masculine sex appeal doesn't start with the jacket; it begins with the skin. From the first layer you put on, you're either building desire or breaking it. Well-fitted briefs that maintain their shape without bunching or sagging. Skin that's clean, smooth, and cared for, not just for looks, but because you respect the vessel you live in. A shirt that frames your chest and shoulders without choking or flaring. Every detail matters.

Women notice everything, not just what you wear but how you wear it. The cut of your tee, the way your pants sit on your hips, the subtle weight of your watch, the placement of your ring, and the blend of your scent. These aren't random fashion choices. They're signals. Strategic tension points. Visual and sensory anchors that whisper: I'm intentional, I'm disciplined, and I'm dangerous in all the right ways.

From base to outerwear, you're telling a story, not about wealth or flash but about control, attention, and sensual presence. Sex appeal isn't loud; it is intentional choices. The man who gets this doesn't chase desire; he triggers it.

Action:

1. Audit your entire outfit, from your underwear to your accessories.

2. Do your pieces fit, feel, and function like they belong to a man with sexual presence?

3. Upgrade one item that's dull, outdated, or neglected.

You Trigger Instant Sexual Dynamics

Sexual dynamics isn't something you force; it's something you trigger. Most women don't respond to noise, performance, or insecurity disguised as bravado. Feminine women respond to energy that's calm, grounded, and unapologetic in its masculinity. The kind that holds space without effort that leads without controlling, and that makes her feel safe to surrender into her natural state.

It's in the restraint, the way your eyes hold hers without blinking first, the way your body doesn't fidget, the way your voice doesn't rise to seek validation, and yes, it's also in your style. Your outfit. Your scent. Your grooming. When a man is composed, precise, and physically dialled in, he amplifies his masculine signal. That signal wakes something in her instantly.

You walk into a space, and her nervous system softens. Her eyes track you without needing a reason. Her posture changes. Not because you perform but because your presence gave her permission to feel. That's dynamics: your calm becomes her surrender. Your discipline becomes her attraction, and your style becomes the visual confirmation that you're exactly who you appear to be.

Action for Today:

1. Before your next interaction with a woman, assess your energy.
2. Are you present, grounded, and leading from stillness, or trying to perform?
3. Adjust one visual layer: your shirt, cologne, watch, or even your walk.
4. Let your presence speak first and let her feel the difference.

March 24th

Masculine Edge in Every Environment

The true mark of a masculine man is not how he performs in a single setting; it's how you carry yourself everywhere. From the gym to the boardroom, from airports to black-tie events, you're always composed, always intentional, and always on point. It's not about overdressing; it's about alignment. Your presence matches the moment without losing your identity.

You don't change who you are to fit the space; you adjust your expression of self with precision. Tailored shorts, clean joggers and a fitted tee in the gym. Crisp denim and clean lines in casual settings. A sharp suit that fits you sharply, people notice. Women feel it. Men respect it.

This level of unity builds elite trust. It tells the world: this man doesn't fake it now, and then you live up to that standard, no matter the environment, and you never show up sloppy, uncertain, or unaligned. Your style, energy, and posture are all unified, and that unity is rare. That unity is power.

March 25th

Stay Lean, Stay Dangerous

Masculine presence isn't about being the biggest guy in the room; it's about being the most capable. Your physique should project readiness, not overcompensation. When your body is lean, mobile, and well-trained, it changes everything: how you move, how you carry yourself, and how your clothes fit your frame. You walk differently. You stand differently. People feel it before they realise it.

A powerful body doesn't need to be oversized; it needs to be efficient. Quick to react. Built to endure and conditioned for pressure with precision strength. The kind of body that moves well under load recovers fast and stays sharp under stress.

Clothes drape better over a trained physique. Movement becomes effortless. You don't need to flex; your presence already signals that you're a warrior. In a world full of men trying to look powerful, the man who moves like he is powerful always stands alone.

Use Eye Contact as a Weapon, not a Wandering Habit

Your eyes speak before your mouth ever does, and a masculine man knows precisely what they're saying. Eye contact isn't a casual habit. It's a weapon. When used intentionally, it becomes one of your most powerful tools. Don't dart around. Don't scan the room. Don't overcommit to an awkward stare. Hold your gaze with calm, grounded control, like you've got nothing to prove and nothing to fear.

Women read emotional safety in your eyes. They scan for certainty. For presence. If you're scattered, distracted, or seeking approval, they feel it instantly. If your eyes are steady, not chasing, just holding, she softens. Her nervous system settles. The dynamics are activated.

Men feel it, too, as a challenge, as quiet dominance. You're not looking through people; you're holding them, and that kind of eye contact creates a sense of space. It changes conversations. It sets the tone. It's the look of a man who sees clearly and leads from a state of stillness, not from a state of performance.

Use it sparingly. Like fire, too much, and you burn the room. Used right, and you own it.

March 27th

You Outclass, Not Compete

A masculine man doesn't walk into a room to compete; he enters to raise the standard. There's a sharp difference between trying to impress and choosing to elevate. You're not seeking the spotlight. You are the energy shift. You walk in clean, intentional, and composed. Your presence doesn't scream, "Look at me." It calmly commands, "Rise with me."

Your style reflects that: fitted, restrained, and minimal. There are no loud patterns and no need for logos—just quiet precision. The cut of your jacket, the fall of your trousers, the weight of your watch, every detail says you live with structure. A polished look conveys that you respect yourself. The silence says you don't chase applause because you already know who you are.

Men take notice, not out of envy, but out of awareness. You move with clarity. Speak with weight. No posturing. No flexing. Just leadership, the kind that doesn't force; it pulls. You remind others, without a word, that they could tighten their standard.

Refinement isn't just attractive; it's magnetic. It speaks of taste, control, and presence. It's not noise; it's a signal.

March 28th

You Radiate "Boss Energy" Everywhere

A masculine man doesn't turn his presence on and off; it's constant. Whether you're grabbing coffee, boarding a flight, walking into the gym, or closing a high-stakes deal, you show up composed, polished, and focused. You don't need to speak first; your posture, grooming, clothing fit, and stillness talk for you.

You look like a man who runs things, not because you say so, but because every detail about you confirms it. The clean edge of your fade. The subtle confidence in your tone. People treat you differently when you move like someone who's already in control—not chasing status but already embodying it, with a presence that opens doors for you, meetings agreed to, and second glances held longer. The world organises itself around you because you're living as someone who expects results, not attention. That's your standard. Boss energy is everywhere.

Action:

1. Before you leave your house for anything, look in the mirror and ask: Would I trust, follow, or invest in this man? If not, adjust.

2. Polish the grooming.

3. Clean the lines.

4. Straighten the posture.

5. Walk into every space like you were born to own it.

You Live as the Standard Other Men Quietly Aspire To

You don't need to announce yourself. You don't need followers. You lead by how you live, and other men notice. They watch your discipline, your style, your sharpness. The way you say less and move more. They may not say it out loud, but they feel it: this is the standard.

While others look for shortcuts, you live by structure. While they chase attention, you build a presence. Your wardrobe is intentional. Your grooming is clean. Your energy is focused. You become the unspoken benchmark, that man other men measure themselves against in silence.

You're not out to impress. You're out to represent, and when every move you make reflects alignment, leadership, and self-respect, it raises the bar for everyone around you without needing to say a word. That's what makes you magnetic. That's what makes you the standard.

Action:

1. Audit your daily behaviour as if someone is watching because they are. One young man. One peer. One silent competitor. Ask: Am I moving like the man I'd admire?

2. Tighten one area: your tone, grooming, schedule, or outfit.

3. Be the man others quietly try to catch up to without ever having to chase.

March 30th

You Attract the Woman You Deserve

When you present yourself as the man who leads with discipline, clarity, and quiet power, you stop attracting women who drain you and start attracting women who respect and respond to you. She isn't drawn just to the clothes you wear but to the energy you embody. She feels your presence when you enter a room, the way your eyes hold hers without flinching, the way your shirt fits with intent, your scent, your silence.

She senses safety without softness, power without arrogance, and certainty without the need to perform; she knows that's rare. That's what feminine women crave: a man who doesn't just take up space but creates structure inside it. When your inner world is connected, and your outer world reflects it, you attract a woman who meets you with respect, softness, and desire, not testing, not control. Masculinity in alignment draws in the feminine without ever needing to chase it.

March 31ˢᵗ

Become the Embodiment of Masculine Style & Presence

It's not about fashion. It's about identity. What we've covered isn't surface; it's structure. From grooming to gait, from tone to tailoring, from energy to execution, every part of you becomes aligned. That alignment is what creates presence. That presence is what defines the highest level of masculine style.

You don't need to raise your voice to be heard. You don't need to dress loud to be seen. You don't need to prove value when your posture, precision, and self-respect already show it. You're built from the inside out, a style that speaks without words, an energy that holds without force, and habits that reflect a man in control.

You've become the standard. The man others watch. The man she feels. The one who doesn't just walk into a room but shifts the energy within it. That's the power of masculine style and presence when it's done right.

Command through consistency. Now, step into it.

April

Fitness & Strength

Build a body that commands respect without needing to say a word

You can't fake strength. You either earn it, or the world exposes your weakness. This section isn't about chasing aesthetics. It's about building a body that aligns with your mission, your mindset, and your message. When your body is sharp, focused, and prepared, it becomes a silent signal of discipline, resilience, and masculine intent.

You don't train for attention; you train for domination. For capability. For the quiet confidence that says, "I can carry the weight. I can take the hit. I won't break." These words aren't about being big. It's about being ready mentally, emotionally, and physically. You are the weapon, and this is your conditioning.

This month, your body becomes a testament to your purpose. Every session reinforces your identity. Every rep teaches you to push when it hurts, focus when it burns, and lead when others stall. Your training becomes your edge, and your physical presence becomes a warning, not a request.

In a world full of talkers, a man with strength doesn't need to say a thing. His presence speaks volumes.

"A strong body isn't for vanity. It's the armour
for a man on a mission."

April 1st

Start with Discipline, Not Motivation

Motivation is unreliable. It fades, it fluctuates, and it lies. Discipline is non-negotiable. A masculine man doesn't wait for the perfect mood or ideal moment; he builds structure and then shows up inside it. Training isn't something you do when it's convenient. It's something you do because it's who you are.

When you lead with discipline, you eliminate the inner noise. You don't ask yourself how you feel; you know that showing up regardless builds momentum. Momentum becomes identity, and identity is what separates men who dabble from men who dominate. You stop skipping. You stop quitting. You stop letting your emotions take control.

Discipline rewires your brain. It tells you: I finish what I start. I show up under pressure. I lead myself before I lead anyone else.

Action:

1. No matter what your schedule looks like, commit to one non-negotiable workout today.
2. Lock it in: time, location, method. Don't wait to "feel it."
3. Show up.

4. Complete it.

5. Log it in your journal or notes with one line: "I didn't wait. I executed."

6. Repeat that enough times, and you won't need motivation ever again.

April 2nd

Discipline Builds Identity

Discipline is the foundation of masculine leadership. It is the quiet force that shapes who you become when no one is watching. When you train without the need for hype, applause, or validation, you start stacking evidence in your mind that you are a man who follows through.

Every rep, every early morning, every time you choose the hard path over the easy one, you are casting a vote for the man you are building. That repetition forms character. Over time, it becomes increasingly complex to distinguish between what you do and who you are. Discipline stops being a task and becomes a standard.

Others begin to see it before you say a word. They trust your leadership because they sense you lead yourself first. You are consistent in a world full of chaos and structured in a culture that rewards shortcuts. That contrast becomes your identity, and it commands respect without needing to ask for it.

April 3rd

Train for Capability, Not Just Looks

A masculine body is not for decoration; it is for domination. Strength that cannot move is useless. A size that cannot last is a wasted effort. You are not training to impress strangers at the gym or get approval on a screen. You are training to be dangerous in the real world.

Build a body that responds under pressure. Focus on the strength that carries, pulls, lifts, and holds. Build mobility that lets you move freely and with power. Develop endurance that allows you to go the distance while others break down. A capable man is prepared for everything, physically and mentally.

When you train for capability, you are not just building muscle; you are forging a weapon. You become reliable, helpful, and respected because you can do what most men only talk about. You do not need to explain it. Your actions, movements, and composure prove it. That is the edge most men will never earn.

Action:

1. Add one functional movement to your training session: carry heavy, short sprints, climb, crawl, or perform a loaded hold.

2. Move your body with purpose, under tension, and outside the frame of the mirror.

3. Build strength you can use, not just admire.

April 4th

Respect the Foundation

Masculine strength isn't built under a barbell; real strength is in the hours no one sees. Your training means nothing if your recovery is weak, your nutrition is sloppy, and your sleep is inconsistent. The strongest men respect the foundation because they understand that discipline outside the gym is what sustains performance inside it.

Sleep is not laziness. It is regeneration. It is hormonal recalibration, nervous system reset, and mental clarity in motion. Hydration is not optional. It affects your focus, endurance, digestion, and recovery. Fuel is not about trends; it's about giving your body what it needs to perform, repair, and thrive.

When you take these three thoughtfully, your body responds with power. Your mind becomes clearer. Your mood sharpens. You stop crashing midday, stop dragging through sessions watching the clock, and start moving like a man built for war, not burnout. These are not minor details. They are the foundation of your performance, presence, and progress. The performance begins long before the workout starts. Start acting like it.

Action:

1. Audit your foundation. How many hours did you sleep last night? How much water have you had today? When was the last time you ate real, quality food?
2. Identify the weakest link and address it before retraining.

April 5th

Recovery Fuels Command

You can't lead when you're depleted. You can't dominate when you're running on fumes. True masculine power requires a sharp mind, a ready body, and controlled emotions, which happen when you prioritise recovery. Sleep, clean fuel, and hydration (like Sodii products with magnesium, sodium, and potassium) are not luxuries. They are weapons.

A man who recovers well thinks more clearly, reacts faster, and carries a presence that others trust. He doesn't overtrain to feed his ego. He trains to stay lethal. Recovery is what gives him the edge. It's the difference between crashing at the first sign of stress or showing up composed when everything else is chaos.

Sacrificing sleep for hustle is amateur and not a man of precision. Ignoring nutrition for convenience is weak. Dehydration kills focus and performance before the first rep. The masculine man honours his health like he honours his word, with discipline and non-negotiable respect.

No breakdown. No burnout. Just sustainable command over yourself. That's what makes you unshakable. That's what makes you trusted. That's what keeps you in the game when others tap out.

April 6th

Master the Basics First

Masculine strength is an important fundamental, not flashy routines or ego-driven complexity. Push. Pull. Squat. Carry. Run. These primal movements are the foundation of real capability. You don't need gimmicks when your body moves like a weapon, with control, power, and efficiency.

Complexity without mastery is weakness dressed up. Men who chase novelty before they've earned the basics expose themselves under pressure. Real masculine presence is grounded in physical literacy, the ability to move well, under load, and with purpose. Master the basics, and you become durable, adaptable, and dangerous.

It's not about looking impressive on social media. It's about being prepared in real life, on uneven ground, under fatigue, in chaos. The man who owns the fundamentals has nothing to prove and everything to deliver. That's where real strength lives, not in performance but in preparation.

Action:

1. Run a full-body fundamentals check.
2. In your next workout, strip it back to one heavy push, one pull, one squat, and one loaded carry.

3. Execute each with perfect form. No ego. Just clean movement under control.

4. You'll know immediately where your real strengths lie and what needs sharpening.

April 7th

Mastery Builds Power

Power isn't how much weight you can lift; it's in how well you move under pressure. Mastery is the invisible edge. It's the sharp line between confidence and recklessness, between true strength and fragile ego.

When you master the basics, you don't just complete movements; you own them. Every push, pull, squat, and carry becomes intentional, efficient, and unshakable. You waste no energy. You move with control. You recover faster, and you dominate the room without needing to draw attention to yourself.

Injury happens when ego outpaces skill. Mastery is what prevents that. It's what keeps you in the game, consistent and respected over the years, not months. The man who moves with mastery doesn't just train harder; he trains smarter. He moves smarter, lasts longer, and leads by example. That's real power: calm, deliberate, and built to last.

April 8th

Lift Heavy, Move Fast, Stay Mobile

A masculine man owns contrast. Strength without speed is limited. Speed without structure is unstable. Mobility without either is soft. You are not sculpting a statue; you are forging a weapon that is lean, explosive, and adaptable.

Lift heavy to build raw force. Move fast to train reaction and command. Stay mobile so your power is engaged at any angle, under pressure, and without hesitation. This contrast is what separates those who are warriors from those who pose as such. Your goal is not bulk; your goal is capacity, the ability to respond with control in any situation.

You are not training to impress; you are training to impress. The man who can sprint, lift, climb, hold, and move cleanly is a man whom others trust and fear, even in silence. Presence comes from preparation, and this is how it's built: through balance, not extremes.

Action:

1. Structure today's session with three elements: one heavy lift, one explosive movement, and one mobility finisher.

2. Example: deadlift, sled push or sprint, then deep lunge holds or rotational stretches.

3. Move like a man who is ready for anything, not just ready to flex.

April 9th

Balanced Power Makes You Dangerous

Real strength is not found solely in size. It is in balance, the ability to generate power, recover quickly, move sharply, and control your body under pressure. When you are lean, fast, and powerful, you become unpredictable. That unpredictability is what makes you dangerous.

You are not one-dimensional. You are not easy to read. You can move, strike, lift, endure, and adapt. That level of balance builds respect without needing to prove anything. Men notice it in how you move. Women feel it in how you hold space. You do not need to raise your voice, flex, or posture. The energy is already there.

You are a threat in the best way, the kind that is composed, capable, and unshakable. It's unnatural to stand still when warriors perform in motion, under load, through chaos. That is what makes people take notice, even in silence.

Action:

1. Choose a training session that includes force, speed, and control.

2. Combine a strength movement, a sprint or explosive drill, and a stability-based finisher.

3. Move with intent, sharp, clean, and calculated.

4. You are not there to compete. You are there to calibrate.

April 10th

Build a Morning Routine That Wins

The way you start your day sets the standard for how you operate. Masculine men don't stumble into the morning reacting to the world; they rise with direction. Your routine is not a ritual of comfort; it's a signal to your mind and body: you lead from the front.

Early training sharpens your mental edge, elevates testosterone levels, activates discipline, and fosters clarity before distractions set in. You are choosing to face resistance before the world even wakes up. That energy permeates everything: your speech, your posture, and your decisions.

You don't need to dominate the entire day in one move; you need to win the first hour. Once you've trained, dialled in, and taken command of your state, you move through life ahead of the curve. You lead, not follow. You act, not react.

Action for Tomorrow Morning:

1. Before your phone, before food, before noise, move.
2. Bodyweight, resistance, or breathwork.
3. Pick one and go all in.

4. Set your tone early.

5. Lock your energy into gear.

6. When the rest of the world hesitates, you've already won round one.

April 11th

Train With Presence

Most men view training as physical effort alone, focusing on weight lifted, distance run, and muscle built. The masculine man who operates at the highest level understands that true mastery of movement doesn't start in the muscles; it begins in the mind and nervous system, and it's refined through the breath.

When you sync your breath with your movement, you're not just oxygenating your blood; you're programming your entire neuromuscular system to fire with precision, force, and control. Inhale with intent before the lift, the strike, the push. Exhale with power as you execute. This breathing pattern signals your body that you're safe, focused, and alert.

You're not just lifting a weight or swinging a hammer; you're anchoring yourself in the now. That connection to breath makes your training a meditation in motion. You're crafting a body that's efficient, intelligent, and lethal. Training to be responsive, not reactive. Grounded and powerful.

April 12th

Hold the Standard in Every Space

Every action, every gesture, every moment reflects your internal structure. How you carry groceries, how you sit at a table, and how you walk into a room —all of it communicates presence.

Strength is not about noise or display. Its posture held with calm command, energy rooted in stillness, movement done with intent. You don't turn it off when the session ends. You don't drop your standards when no one is looking. The man you are under load should be the man you are in daily life.

Masculine energy doesn't clock out. It sharpens through repetition, precision, and holding yourself accountable in the most minor details because how you do anything reflects how you do everything.

Action:

1. Pick one moment you usually overlook: how you get out of the car, how you sit in a chair, how you walk into a store.
2. Slow down, correct your posture, and move with intention.
3. No slouching, no dragging.
4. Let your presence precede your voice.

April 13th

Being Lean Shows Discipline

Staying lean is not about vanity; it is about visible control. It reflects restraint, consistency, and sharp decision-making. When a man is lean, it tells the world he governs what goes into his body, how he moves it, and when he rests. He does not drift through his days; he calculates.

Being lean doesn't happen by accident. It developed through habit, clarity, and standards that most are not willing to uphold. It means you don't eat to feel good; you eat to perform. You don't train for approval; you train for an edge.

A lean body signals purpose. It's about being the most capable, the most prepared, and the most focused. People see it before you speak. Women feel it before you touch it. Men register it without needing to be told. It's the mark of a warrior who respects himself enough to stay sharp and dangerous.

April 14th

Primal Power

A masculine man doesn't wait for the perfect environment to train. He doesn't need polished floors, air-conditioned gyms, or mirrors to measure progress. Strength, for him, is not a luxury or a hobby; it's a primal requirement. When you understand that, you stop making excuses. You train wherever you stand. You turn the world into your gym.

Flip a tyre. Swing a sledgehammer. Carry a log. Climb a rope. These movements connect you to a raw and functional strength. It's not about isolating a muscle; it's about integrating your body, breath, and grit into one unified act of power.

There's no excuse not to train when you understand the importance of this. Mother Earth provides the resistance. When you operate in this manner, you not only become physically stronger, but your mental strength also explodes to new levels.

The masculine man doesn't need permission to become powerful. He creates it with his own two hands, one rep at a time.

April 15th

Pain Trains the Mind

Pain is not punishment; it is a form of programming. Every time you choose discomfort in training, you train your nervous system to remain calm in the face of pressure. You teach your mind to hold steady while your body struggles. That's where the masculine edge is forged, not in comfort but in control through chaos.

Masculine men don't avoid pain; they seek it with intent. They know that daily suffering under their terms makes life's tests feel lighter. When you've already faced the storm in training, nothing external has the power to break you. Pain becomes familiar. Challenge becomes a trigger for focus, not fear.

Here's where discipline meets precision: train in odd numbers. Most people stop on even numbers, such as 10 reps, 12 reps, or 20 minutes. Why? Men are wired to finish on a number that feels clean and complete. That's precisely why you don't. Push past that internal quit point. Five reps. Nine. Eleven. One more than you think. One more than the guy next to you. Not for ego but for discipline. That extra rep is the rep that builds the mindset no one else has.

Pain sharpens. Precision refines. Discipline separates.

Action:

1. Whatever your reps were going to be, add one. And make it odd.
2. Finish your sets at 5, 11, or 15.
3. The final rep is not for the muscle. It's for your mind.
4. Do it and walk away knowing you're not programmed; you're in command.

April 16th

Train Like It's Life, not a Hobby

You are not the average man who squeezes in three workouts a week and rewards himself with junk on Sunday. You're not clocking in and out of your discipline. You are building a body and a mind that hold the line every day.

Training is not something you do; it's a reflection of who you are. Your body is your operating system. Your training is your calibration. If your routine looks like a hobby, your results will reflect it. When your training becomes a non-negotiable extension of your identity, everything changes. You walk into every room with a presence. People feel it before you speak.

You move like an athlete. You recover like a professional. You build a structure around your output and your rest. You track progress. You train when it's raining when you're tired, and no one's watching. That's how a masculine man builds dominance. Quiet, calculated, consistent.

This level of discipline spills into every area: how you handle pressure, how you communicate, and how you lead. You're not just strong in the gym. You're composed in chaos, efficient under fatigue, and calm when others fold. That doesn't come from the part-time effort. It comes from a full-time identity.

Action:

1. Audit your current training and recovery practices.
2. Is it built for dominance or convenience?
3. Tighten your structure.
4. Set your training days, sleep targets, recovery windows, and meals like you're preparing for battle, not the beach.
5. Move as if your life depends on it.

April 17th

Lifestyle Creates Legacy

Fitness isn't a phase, a trend, or a temporary fix. It's your lifestyle, and that lifestyle becomes your legacy. How you move, how you eat, how you recover, and how you carry yourself daily sets the tone for the men around you and the generations that follow.

You don't train hard one week and vanish the next. You don't eat clean only when it's easy. You live the standard day in, day out, whether eyes are on you or not. That consistency is what makes you reliable. That reliability is what earns respect.

People follow those who are living it, not those who talk about becoming it. When you embody discipline with precision and patience, your results have a ripple effect. You influence without effort, you lead without asking, and you leave a mark without needing applause.

Your body becomes a symbol, not just of strength, but of self-respect. Your routine becomes a framework others try to replicate. Your presence becomes a benchmark, not in what you say but in how you live every single day. That's legacy.

April 18th

Your Body Becomes a Visual Standard

Before you say a word, your body speaks with clarity. It says this man shows up. This man has standards. This man doesn't negotiate from a position of weakness. It tells the world that you put in work, not for praise, but because it's who you are.

A strong, lean, well-built physique is not just aesthetics; it's discipline on display. It signals control over impulse, commitment under pressure, and a lifestyle rooted in self-respect. You don't need to prove anything when your posture, symmetry, and energy already carry the message: this man is built, not gifted.

Your presence becomes the measuring stick, not because you're chasing admiration but because you've become a testament to what living up to the standard looks like. In a world full of talk, your body shows the receipts.

Action:

1. Take a full-body photo in a neutral stance, with no flex, no posing, just presence.
2. Look at it with honesty.
3. Ask yourself: Does this reflect the man I claim to be?

4. Adjust your training and lifestyle accordingly based on the answer.

5. This isn't about judgment; it's about alignment. You are the standard now. Start moving like it.

April 19th

Masculine Shape Triggers Biological Attraction

You can say all the right things. You can be kind, intelligent, even successful. None of it cuts through faster than how your body looks walking into a room. That V-shaped frame, broad shoulders, narrow waist, strong chest, and back are primal coding, hardwired into human biology as a marker of health, strength, and dominance.

Women don't analyse this consciously; they feel it. The structure of your body speaks before your voice does. Broad shoulders signal protection. A solid chest and back suggest the power to defend. A tight waist shows discipline and vitality. Your body shape becomes a visual declaration of leadership, capability and security.

From an evolutionary standpoint, this V-taper shape serves as a beacon of virility and status. In ancient tribes, that shape meant that man hunted, fought, built, and survived. In modern life, it still speaks, just in a more refined language. In the club, on the beach, walking into a boardroom, when your frame is sharp, your presence is amplified.

You don't need to be the biggest man in the room. You need to be the most proportional and intentional. That's the edge. Women may not always remember what you said, but they'll never forget how your silhouette made them feel. That's attraction without effort. That's the power of masculine structure.

April 20th

Dominance Is Felt, Not Spoken

Absolute dominance isn't loud. It doesn't need to convince. A man who is physically trained, mentally clear, and emotionally still walks into a room and shifts the atmosphere without saying a word. Your posture is tall but relaxed. Your eye contact is steady, not aggressive. Your movements are precise, controlled, and unfazed by the chaos around you.

You're the kind of man who doesn't posture, boast, or seek validation. You lead yourself, and that presence commands others without needing to raise your voice. Women feel safe around you and captivated by your energy. Masculine dominance is not about intimidation; it's about grounded certainty. You become the still point in a spinning room. The calm in a storm. The man others feel before they even see.

The body reinforces this. When training is a part of your daily life, your chest sits open, your spine is aligned, your gait is smooth, and your nervous system is regulated. Your very presence says I'm in control of myself and, if necessary, of this moment. That's what makes women lean in and men take notice.

Action:

1. Walk into every space today with calm, grounded energy.
2. Shoulders back, chin neutral, chest open, breath slow.
3. Make eye contact deliberately.
4. Hold it just long enough to show presence, then move on.
5. Let your presence speak before you act. Dominance doesn't shout. It anchors.

April 21st

Strength Creates Sexual Confidence

Strength isn't just for the gym; it's the foundation of how you show up in every intimate moment. Train to move under load, endure discomfort, and maintain form under fatigue. That doesn't disappear when the weights are racked. It carries over straight into the bedroom.

A strong man has control of rhythm, breath, pressure, and tempo. You're not panicked or hurried. You're grounded. Your stamina strengthens through reps, and your confidence isn't performative; it's owned. Women sense it. They relax into it because your physical capability becomes their emotional safety.

When you know your body can go the distance, lift her with ease, change angles with power, or hold tension without collapsing, it changes how you move. You're not overthinking. You're leading. You're fully present. You become the kind of lover she doesn't forget because the masculine edge that built your body now meets her in the deepest place.

Action:

1. Train your body to perform under tension and sustain control, just like in sex.

2. Use tempo reps: slow eccentrics, controlled pauses, explosive drive.

3. Do a 3-second descent, 2-second pause, and controlled lift.

4. Whether it's push-ups, squats, or weighted carries, you're not just building muscle; you're programming sexual precision.

April 22nd

Strength Equals Reliability

Strength isn't just about lifting weights; it's about being the man she can lean on when everything else feels uncertain. A trained, capable body is more than impressive; it's reassuring. When you move with power and steadiness, when you can lift her effortlessly, carry her through the chaos, and stand firm when things get messy, she feels it in her nervous system.

Strength tells her she's safe. Not only physically but also emotionally. If you take care of your body with precision, you're likely to take care of her with intention. You become the consistent one who doesn't fold under pressure and who doesn't disappear when things get tough.

Masculine strength is more than a gym flex. It's the quiet promise behind every touch, every held door, every moment you ground your woman's energy without needing to fix it. That's what creates deep trust. That's what opens the door to real intimacy, where she doesn't just want you; she chooses to surrender to you.

April 23rd

Muscle is Armour, But Mobile is Useful Armour

Real masculine strength isn't stiff, oversized, or showy. It's functional. Mobile. Reactive. You don't train to look big in photos. You train to move like a lion, lean, powerful, coiled with purpose.

Muscle without movement is dead weight. When you're agile, explosive, and fluid, your body becomes both armour and invitation. You can lift, sprint, rotate, carry, climb, and still walk with the kind of relaxed control that women feel instantly. They don't crave mass; they crave mastery. The way you stretch, move and take up space without tension lets her know you're in full command.

There's a magnetism in a man who's strong yet effortlessly mobile. It says: I can protect, I can perform, I can move through chaos with precision. That's what triggers primal attraction. You become both the safe place and the thrill: the grounded force and the wild edge.

The men who dominate aren't the biggest; they're the most capable.

Action for Today:

1. Incorporate movement-based strength training: kettlebell flows, Turkish get-ups, weighted carries, and animal crawls.

2. Add 10 minutes of mobility drills post-workout: hips, ankles, spine.

3. Build strength that moves, not just a muscle that flexes.

April 24th

Testosterone Becomes Your Ally

Heavy lifts, explosive movement, deep sleep, and sunlight. When you train like a man, recover like a pro, and eat with intention, your testosterone levels naturally rise, and that changes everything.

Higher testosterone isn't just about libido. It sharpens your thinking. It deepens your voice. It improves your posture. It makes your presence thicker, more grounded, more unshakable. You feel less anxious and more assertive. Less reactive and more decisive. You walk through the world with your chest open and your mind transparent. You stop questioning yourself. You move.

Women sense that primal charge, the quiet heat that says you're not just showing up; you're ready to lead. Testosterone makes your masculinity felt before it's spoken.

Action:

1. Lift heavy, compound movements only (squat, deadlift, overhead press).
2. Sprint hard, 4 to 6 rounds of 20 seconds max effort.
3. Recover and get 8+ hours of deep, uninterrupted sleep.
4. Cut out sugar, seed oils, and alcohol for at least 48 hours.
5. Let your biology do its job. Let your edge sharpen from the inside out.

April 25th

You Handle Her Energy with Strength, Not Fragility

Feminine energy is wild, emotional, reactive, and powerful. Most men collapse under it because they're untrained, physically weak, emotionally scattered, and mentally unclear. When you're a man with strength in your frame and stillness in your mind, you become the container, not the casualty.

You don't flinch when she tests you. You don't react when her emotions spike. You stay grounded, present, and calm, not cold, but immovable. That's what makes her feel safe. That's what makes her open. Feminine energy craves a masculine presence strong enough to absorb the storm without trying to silence it.

That's where the real attraction is born. When a woman senses that she can let go in conversation, in conflict, in bed, because you can hold it all. She doesn't have to manage your emotions or filter her truth. She can surrender. In that surrender comes explosive chemistry, deeper trust, and sex that transcends performance because she's no longer holding back.

Be the man who can handle her, and that starts by building yourself, not just in body but in presence.

Action:

1. Next time tension rises, in an argument, a heated moment, or an emotional intensity, pause.
2. Breathe.
3. Hold your posture.
4. Let a woman's energy move, but don't match it.
5. Don't shrink, fix, or flee.
6. Ground yourself like a mountain.
7. That's the moment she feels he can hold me.

April 26th

Clean Body, Dirty Intent, in the Best Way

You walk in smelling fresh, with smooth skin and sharp hair. Your grooming is immaculate, not to impress, but because it reflects your discipline. Everything about you is clean, composed, and elevated. Underneath that polished exterior, there's an edge. There's hunger. There's intent.

Masculine energy isn't about being reckless; it's about being ready. You don't wear vulgarity on your sleeve, but your presence carries something raw beneath the surface. It's in your stillness. Your eyes. The way you move close and slow, unbothered but always in control. She knows you won't just protect her; you'll take her. When the moment's right.

That dynamic is electric. Clean Signals Care. Dirty signals depth. When you fuse the two, when you show up well-groomed with that warrior look behind your eye, she can't help but wonder what it would be like to let go in your arms. It's not what you say. It's what you withhold. That restraint is magnetic.

Action:

1. Refine your ritual.

2. Cold Shower.

3. Use a high-quality exfoliant.

4. Apply oil or lotion, not for softness, but to keep your skin clean and healthy.

5. Pick a cologne that lingers without overpowering (Tom Ford Oud Wood or Creed Aventus).

6. Walk through your day like a man who could be anyone's calm or anyone's storm.

April 27th

Your Endurance Becomes Her Freedom

Endurance isn't just about running further or lasting longer in the gym; it's about what kind of man you are when things stretch, burn, or break down, and women feel it. If she senses that your energy fades quickly, your mind checks out under pressure, or your body gives in when things get real, she'll never fully let go. To surrender, she must know you won't.

When you're built with depth, physically conditioned, emotionally present, and mentally locked in, she relaxes into you. She stops testing and holding back because you've shown her that her emotions won't overwhelm you. Her body won't exhaust you. Life won't pull you under.

Whether it's during a storm, a crisis, or in the middle of the night when she wants all of you, if you're the man who can go the distance, she'll give you more of herself. The deeper she trusts your endurance, the more powerful the intimacy becomes. The better the sex. The bolder the connection.

She doesn't want a man who performs. She wants a man who lasts. That doesn't come from theory. It comes from training your body, disciplining your breath, and sharpening your focus. You don't quit early. You don't need breaks. You hold the line.

That's what allows her to melt. That's what makes her crave only you.

Action:

1. Test your endurance, both physically and mentally.
2. Choose one workout: AMRAP (as many rounds as possible in 20 minutes), long-distance run, or heavy circuit with minimal rest.
3. No music.
4. No breaks.
5. Just presence and breath.
6. Push past the point where most stop.

April 28th

Self-Mastery Becomes Sexual Mastery

Every time you say no to junk food, complete the complex set or resist the urge to take the easy option, you're wiring control into your nervous system. That same control is evident when it matters most: in intimacy. The way you master your body in discipline becomes the way you master it in desire.

Sexual confidence doesn't come from experience; it comes from control. From being able to slow things down, stay present, read your partner, guide her, and not be run by impulse. When cravings in daily life rule a man, he becomes ruled by them in bed. That leads to selfishness, speed, and disappointment. When you've trained yourself to delay gratification, focus under pressure, and breathe through intensity, that mastery transfers into the bedroom.

You last longer, connect deeper and lead better. Your energy doesn't scatter. Your attention doesn't fade. You build tension, release it with precision, and command the pace. Sex with a man who's trained in restraint and presence isn't a performance; it's an experience.

You don't chase pleasure. You build it. You earn it. You own it.

Action:

1. Pick one craving you usually give in to: sugar, screen time, comfort, and deny it.

2. Replace it with something that strengthens you: a cold shower, 50 push-ups, or a walk-in silence.

3. Train that inner muscle. It's the same one that makes you unforgettable between the sheets.

April 29th

Your Body Becomes a Portal to Her Fantasy

Most men chase validation. You embody the vision. You become the man she imagined, but she has almost given up on finding. The one who doesn't just look the part but moves the part. Lean, powerful, and still within. A body shaped by intention. A presence that says nothing yet commands everything.

When you've built through discipline, not just aesthetics, your body radiates something she can't ignore. You walk into a room, and she feels you. Not because you're loud but because of your shape, your energy, and your stillness; they all speak of control, purpose, and danger wrapped in your presence.

You don't need to pose. You don't need to talk big. You don't even need to initiate. You exist in complete alignment, and that ignites curiosity. When a woman sees your physique, your scent, and your eyes, she starts to imagine her fantasies with you. When you finally touch her, it's not a physical moment; it's the release of everything she hoped a man could be.

She feels the edge. She feels the command. Most importantly, she feels the devotion underneath it. The man who disciplines his body, who restrains his energy, who doesn't scatter himself for the world, is the man who chooses her with full presence.

That's the kind of experience she remembers in silence and years later, wondering if she'll ever feel it again.

Action:

1. Move like the man she dreams about.
2. Train for presence, not just appearance.
3. Hold eye contact with stillness.
4. Groom for sharpness.
5. Walk into a room today; don't search for attention; pull it through quiet command. Let your body do the talking.

April 30th

You Don't Just Look Like a Man; you Live as One

Your physique reflects your discipline. Your presence reflects your inner command. Your touch reflects your restraint, and your energy speaks before your words ever do.

You've become the man who doesn't try to be masculine; you are masculine. Every detail, every habit, every rep, every decision stacks into the man who walks into the room and doesn't need to prove anything. You've sculpted your body to reflect your purpose. You've trained your nervous system to stay grounded under pressure. You've built a style and presence that turns heads without ever needing to ask for attention.

Women feel it, the safety, the power, the danger. Men notice it: the discipline, the edge, the standard. Most of all, you feel it. That certainty. That locked-in sense of "I'm exactly who I say I am."

Becoming a masculine man isn't about building strength; it's about embodying it. From your posture to your presence, from your breath to your bedroom, you've created a sacred unity, and that's not common. That's elite status.

You don't just carry masculine energy; you've mastered it. You've become the man others admire, women crave, and you trust. That's what this is all about. Self-mastery. Walking as a masculine man, built, not born.

May

Trust & Honour

Be the man whose name is spoken with respect, even when you're not in the room.

Your reputation is your shadow; it follows you everywhere, even when you're not present. This month is about becoming the man whose name carries weight, whose word carries value, and whose actions speak long after you're gone. Trust and Honour aren't buzzwords. They're currency, and as a masculine man, you either build that currency daily or you go broke trying to fake it.

You don't need to prove yourself when your word already has a track record. You don't need to convince anyone when your presence holds consistency. Honour isn't about being liked; it's about being respected by men, trusted by women, and feared by anything weak within yourself.

This month is about eliminating the gaps between who you say you are and how you live. It's about living with such integrity that your decisions remain consistent, regardless of your mood, audience, or outcome. You say it, you do it. You promise it, you deliver it. You live it, you lead it.

When you become the person people know they can count on, you stop chasing status and start building a legacy.

"Your word is your spine. If it bends,
everything collapses."

Make Promises Sparingly, Keep Them Relentlessly

A masculine man doesn't hand out commitments as easily as he hands out compliments. You know every promise is a contract, and your name, reputation, and identity are on the line with every word.

A man of trust and honour speaks with precision. He commits rarely, but when he does, you can carve it in stone.

Your word is your brand in relationships, in business, in brotherhood. If you say you'll show up, you show up. If you say you've got it handled, do it. That consistency becomes magnetic. Women feel safer. Men respect you more, and you respect yourself deeply because you're not chasing approval; you're protecting your standard.

Masculine power isn't loud; it's reliable. That's the difference. When your name is mentioned, people should say, "If he said it, it's done." That's the kind of man people trust with opportunities, with leadership, and with their lives.

People Trust You Before You Speak

When you live with ruthless consistency, doing what you say, finishing what you start, and showing up without excuses, people feel your presence before you open your mouth. That's earned power. You don't need to convince, posture, or sell yourself. Your reputation speaks. Your energy confirms it.

The quiet dominance of a man is what makes him undeniable. You've become so reliable, so dialled in, so exact in how you move that others instinctively know: this is a man I can trust. He won't fold under pressure. He doesn't need applause. He delivers.

Your name alone will open doors. Not from noise, from the authority behind your choices. Whether in business, in brotherhood, or in intimacy, people feel safer, more precise, and sharper in your presence. You don't just talk the part; you've lived it. Repeatedly. Until your character becomes a signal, not just a trait.

Action:

1. Audit your daily integrity.
2. Choose one task you've been avoiding or postponing and complete it to perfection today.

3. Say nothing.

4. Let your completion speak for itself. One act of follow-through, done without show, builds more trust than a thousand promises.

5. Power doesn't announce itself; it arrives. So should you.

May 3rd

Treat Your Word Like Currency

Your word is a form of capital, and every time you speak, you're either investing in your value or bleeding it dry. Masculine men understand this. They don't bluff. They don't talk just to be heard. When they speak, it's because something needs to be said, and when they commit, they follow through with militant precision.

Every loose promise, every white lie, every time you exaggerate or try to impress, it's like handing out counterfeit money. People may take it once, but they'll never trust you again. Your credibility fades, and without credibility, you've got nothing.

When you move in silence and act with sharp intent, you build equity. You become a man others trust to lead, to protect, to perform. Your word starts to carry weight, not because you talk often, but because you talk with purpose.

Masculine men speak less, mean more, and follow through relentlessly. They build value with every word they don't say and back every word they do. Over time, that becomes an unshakable power.

Your voice is an investment. Speak like you're building a legacy.

May 4th

Never Lie to Yourself

You can lie to others and walk away untouched, but lie to yourself, and everything collapses. That's the crack in the foundation no one sees until the whole thing falls. A masculine man doesn't fear the truth. He seeks it, no matter how brutal, because clarity is a form of power.

Self-deception is how weak men stay comfortable. They avoid mirrors, justify shortcuts, and pretend they're doing their best, knowing deep down they're not. A man of Honour calls his bluff. He confronts his excuses. He breaks the illusion, not his word.

Trust doesn't start with others; it begins internally. If you can't believe your voice, why should anyone else? Masculine strength develops through ruthless self-awareness. That's how you sharpen your edge and stay aligned.

Action:

1. Write down one lie you've been telling yourself about your discipline, your effort, and your standards.
2. Write the truth next to it in clear language.
3. No fluff. Just facts.

4. Read it out loud. Feel the sting.

5. Now decide to live with the lie or rise with the truth.

6. This is how men rebuild inner trust, one hard truth at a time.

May 5th

Your Leadership Is Quiet, But Absolute

Masculine leadership doesn't need noise. It doesn't need barking, flexing, or chasing obedience. It leads through certainty, as evident in the way you walk into a room, the way you make decisions and the way you handle adversity. When you carry yourself with unshakable clarity, people feel it before they hear it.

You don't need to force anyone to follow. You move with such grounded conviction that others naturally align with you. Your tone is calm, your standards are sharp, and your actions are consistent. That's the kind of leadership that doesn't demand respect; it draws it.

Quiet leadership is the highest form of masculine command. You don't need a spotlight. You don't need validation. You move, and the room shifts.

May 6th

Say No Without Guilt

Masculine men do not say yes to avoid discomfort. They say yes when it aligns with their mission, values, and purpose. Anything else is a distraction, and distractions drain your power. Every "yes" given to please someone is a "no" to your progress.

Protect your time, energy, and presence as if they were sacred because they are. You only get so many hours, so many deep work blocks, and so many clear windows to train, lead, and build. Waste them on appeasing others, and you dilute your edge.

Your power is in your selectivity. Your "no" isn't rude; it's refined. It communicates that your life is focused and not available for rent.

Action:

1. Say no to one thing you would usually accept out of guilt, a meeting, a favour, or a task that dilutes your direction.
2. Do it clearly and calmly, without explanation or apology.
3. Reclaim that time and put it into something that sharpens you.
4. Saying no to the unnecessary is saying yes to the man you're becoming.

May 7th

Show Up, Especially When You Don't Feel Like It

Anyone can train when conditions are favourable. Anyone can lead when they're inspired. But the days when you're tired, unfocused, and frustrated are the proving ground.

Masculine men don't operate from emotion; they operate from a sense of commitment. You know, every time you show up when it's inconvenient, you're stacking evidence. That evidence becomes confidence, and that confidence becomes trust, the kind of trust people can feel before you even speak.

The world doesn't need another man who shows up when it's fun. It needs the man who shows up when it's necessary. That's the man others rely on. That's the man women feel safe with. That's the man who builds a legacy, not just momentum.

Action:

1. Pick one thing you don't feel like doing today: your workout, your project, your network outreach, or your early wake-up.
2. Do it anyway. Do it with focus. No shortcuts. No pity.

3. Mark it mentally or on paper.

4. That's a win few will see, but you will feel. Stack enough of those, and your character becomes unbreakable.

May 8th

You Become the Benchmark

You're not out to impress. You're out to live aligned. That alignment between your values, words, actions, and energy becomes rare. Unmistakable. Masculine. That's when you stop being one of many and become the benchmark.

Other men might not say it out loud, but they notice. They study how you move. The way you handle setbacks. The way you don't react emotionally. The way you walk into a room without needing to prove anything because your presence already proves everything. They compare themselves to you, not because you brag, but because your consistency exposes their excuses.

It all starts with self-trust. You trust your decisions because you show up daily, even when it's uncomfortable. You don't lie to yourself, and that internal trust becomes a force. It's visible. Palpable. You become the man others instinctively trust, with leadership, responsibility, women, and truth.

That's power. That's not gifted, and when your life becomes a reflection of that trust and alignment, others start adjusting to your standard.

You don't copy anyone. You don't compete with anyone. You live so clearly and so sharply that others have no choice but to measure themselves against you.

That's when you know you've become the benchmark.

May 9th

Your Presence Feels Like Home and Fire

A masculine man embodies two forces simultaneously: stability and intensity. He's grounded like a fortress but carries a fire behind his eyes that commands attention. That duality is rare. It's why women feel both safe and electrified in your space. Your calm isn't passive; it's powerful. Your fire isn't chaos; it's controlled purpose.

She leans into your energy because she can trust it. There's no guessing. No performance. Just presence. That presence is earned, built through self-trust, discipline, and showing up in full command of yourself.

You don't just say you're dependable. You live it. That's why people relax when you're in the room. It's why she lets her walls down because you've mastered yourself. You're not seeking attention. You're anchoring the room. You're the home she never had and the danger she craves, all in one.

Action:

1. Slow down.
2. Walk, speak, and make eye contact with deliberate intent.

3. Let your stillness carry weight.

4. Speak less but with more purpose.

5. In every interaction today, carry the thought: "I am both safety and spark." That's what trust and Honour feel like to you and her.

Tell the Truth, Even When It Costs You

Masculine men don't bend the truth to please people. They speak the truth because it's the backbone of trust with others and within themselves. When you tell the truth, especially when it stings, you send a signal: I don't fold to pressure. My actions aren't for comfort. My actions are for clarity.

Anyone can be honest when there are no consequences. It's when truth threatens your ego, your image, or your advantage that the test is on. That's where men of Honour rise because they'd rather lose a moment of approval than carry the weight of dishonesty.

Women feel it. Men respect it, and most importantly, you trust yourself more with every attempt. You know you won't sell your integrity to make someone else feel better. That sharpens your masculine edge. That builds a presence others can't fake.

Action:

1. Call out one area where you've been avoiding the whole truth with someone else or with yourself.
2. Write it.
3. Speak it directly, calmly, and without justification.

4. Let the discomfort sharpen you because every time you choose truth over ease, your presence becomes more trusted, more respected, and more undeniably masculine.

May 11th

Defend What You Value

A masculine man doesn't just talk about values; he defends them. Quietly. Consistently. Unshakably. In a world that rewards conformity, softness, and neutrality, you draw precise lines, not with aggression but with conviction. You know what you stand for and, more importantly, what you won't tolerate.

If you don't protect your principles, they're not values; they're just ideas. Your honour, your code and your way of living are of high value, not just preached. When you stand for something real, you will be tested. People will push. Situations will tempt. If you flinch, everything crumbles.

When you don't, when you speak with weight, act with precision, and follow through without apology, people feel it. They may disagree with you, but they respect you. Women feel safer around you. Men trust your leadership, and you trust your backbone.

Action:

1. Identify one value that matters to you: discipline, loyalty, truth, whatever it is, and set a boundary around it.

2. Enforce it today.

3. Say nowhere you'd usually fold.

4. Speak up when you usually stay silent.

5. Stand firm. One act of defence sharpens the entire frame.

6. Masculinity isn't loud; it's an unbreakable alignment.

May 12th

Be Respected Behind Closed Doors

You know you're a man of Honour not by the noise made in your presence but by the silence that speaks when you're not in the room. People trust you. They reference your name with respect. You don't just perform when eyes are on you; you live your standard whether anyone's watching or not.

You keep your word. You stay consistent. You always show up sharp and solid. Over time, that builds something most men never earn: a reputation. Not hype. Not charisma. Character.

Your name carries weight. Quietly. Cleanly. Behind closed doors, people don't need to guess who you are; they already know. You've proven it. Through follow-through. Through truth. Through every decision that could have been easier but wasn't.

That's the mark of masculine trust. Not just presence, proof. You don't just talk like a man of Honour. You live like one, and the world remembers.

May 13th

Do the Right Thing, Not the Easy Thing

You are tested when the stakes are high, when the easy way out is right in front of you, whispering, "Nobody will know." But you will know, and that's what separates you from the masses.

When everything's on the line — money, reputation, relationship, advantage — most men fold. They rationalise, cut corners, and justify weakness. But a man of Honour stands firm. You don't just know what's right; you choose it, especially when it comes at a cost. Especially when it's inconvenient, that's the battle between impulse and integrity, and masculine men win that war daily.

Honour isn't just an idea; it's an operating system. It shows in how you speak about others when they're not present. How do you handle temptation when no one's watching? How do you take accountability when you could easily pass the blame? You hold the line because if you don't, no one else will.

It's in your energy, your restraint, and your backbone. There's safety in knowing you won't betray your code, even in the face of adversity. That's not just attractive; it's magnetic. It's rare. It builds the kind of respect that lasts.

You're not here to be a people pleaser. You're here to be trusted.

Action:

1. Think of one decision you've been avoiding, one that would be easy to cut a corner on.
2. Face it head-on today.
3. Take the path that protects your integrity, not your comfort. Speak the uncomfortable truth.
4. Complete the task without taking shortcuts.
5. Be the man who chooses hard because it's right, not convenient because it's easy.

May 14th

Your Boundaries Attract, Not Repel

Masculine presence isn't about being agreeable; it's about being clear and direct. When you hold firm boundaries, people don't see you as rigid. They see you as trustworthy. They know where you stand, and that gives them certainty, the kind most men are too afraid to provide.

Weak men often say yes to everything and wonder why they're overlooked, disrespected, or taken advantage of. Masculine men say no with clarity and calm. You don't explain. You don't justify. You honour your line. That line becomes a signal to women, to peers, to the world that this is a man who values his time, his energy, and his principles.

Women are attracted to men with transparent edges. Your boundary says, "This is what I tolerate. This is what I protect." That creates safety. That creates polarity. In a culture of blurred lines and soft speech, it's your boundaries that make you unforgettable.

You're not here to please everyone. You're here to command respect, magnetise truth, and lead by example. Boundaries aren't barriers; they're invitations to step up or step aside, and when you live by them, you stop chasing approval and start attracting alignment.

Trust is Earned Daily, With Yourself First

Masculine trust doesn't start in the boardroom, the bedroom, or the battlefield; it begins in the mirror. You either keep the promises you make to yourself, or you teach your mind you're full of noise. Every time you hit snooze, skip the workout, avoid the conversation, or delay the mission, you lose a piece of your respect.

That's the truth most men run from. They want others to believe in them before they've earned their own belief. It doesn't work that way. Confidence, presence, and leadership are all built on evidence. That evidence is collected in silence, long before anyone is watching.

You said you'd train. Did you?

You said you'd cut the excuses. Did you?

You said you'd level up. Are you showing up or just talking?

The masculine man wakes up and does what he said he'd done yesterday. Not because it's easy but because it's necessary. That's where trust begins. That's what people feel when you're in their presence. That's the edge you carry that makes you different and respected.

Action:

1. Write down three things you committed to doing today: fitness, food, business, and mindset.
2. No fluff.
3. No, maybe.
4. At the end of the day, check them off or own that you didn't. You're either reinforcing trust or sabotaging it.
5. Your identity is being shaped, rep by rep, word by word. Build the man who follows through. That's the man others follow.

May 16th

Your Energy Dominates Without Intimidating

Real masculine power isn't loud, aggressive, or performative; it's undeniable. You walk into a room, and people take notice, not because you're trying to stand out but because you're grounded and anchoring, composed, precise, and confident. That steadiness is rare, and in a world full of noise, it becomes magnetic.

You don't posture. You don't flex. You just are, and being grounded in truth, discipline, and self-respect creates a presence that shifts the room. Your eye contact, tone, and calm all speak louder than words ever could.

Masculine men lead through stillness, not struggle. Through truth, not tactics. You don't dominate to overpower; you dominate by being fully aligned. No masks. No desperation. Just strength lived and felt.

May 17th

Be the Rock, Not the Ripple

Masculine energy doesn't flinch. It doesn't get pulled into chaos, dragged by moods, or thrown off course by opinions. The masculine man is the anchor, steady, composed, and unmoved, while the world reacts, complains, and spirals out of control.

When others get emotional, you stay clear. When situations get loud, you remain calm. When things go sideways, you lead. Not because you're suppressing your emotions but because you've learned to master them. You feel it, but it doesn't control you. That control isn't cold; it's power. It's what allows you to show up consistently, speak with clarity, and handle high-pressure situations.

Your woman feels it. She leans into your roundedness because it gives her freedom to flow. The world feels it. Your presence becomes a stabiliser in unstable environments. While everyone else ripples with whatever energy hits them, you remain the rock, unshaken, clear, and always aligned.

You don't ride the current. You become the shoreline waves crash against and respect.

You Become a Man of Depth, Not an Image

Most men chase attention. You build substance. While others project filtered strength, you live the kind that doesn't need explaining; it's felt. You don't need approval because your word, your actions, and your values already align. That consistency creates gravity. You're not a performance; you're a presence.

You're not trying to be "the man"; you are the man because you've earned every inch of yourself. You've confronted your shadow, refined your standards, and chosen consistency over convenience.

Women don't want you to be perfect. They want you real. A man who stands in truth, not trends. A man whose yes means yes and whose presence says more than words ever could. That kind of man doesn't fade after the first impression. He deepens, layer by layer, moment by moment, and that's what makes him unforgettable.

Action:

1. Audit yourself.
2. Take one aspect of your life, relationships, health, and business, and ask: Does how I show up match who I say I am? If not, adjust.
3. Sharpen your edge where it has dulled.
4. Speak less, align more.
5. Let today's actions reinforce your depth, not your image.

You Leave a Legacy of Strength, Not Scars

Masculine men think beyond the moment. You're not here to impress for the day; you're here to leave a mark that outlives you. Every choice, every word, every boundary you set either builds a legacy or leaves damage. The man of Honour knows this, so he moves with precision.

You don't lead through force. You lead through consistency. Through truth. Through presence. The women you connect with feel safer, not more guarded. The men you influence rise, not shrink. You're not someone they have to recover from; you're someone they remember because you made them better.

Strength, when aligned with trust, becomes a legacy. You build stronger families. Sharper teams. Partners are more grounded.

A masculine man doesn't just carry muscle or money but meaning. The power that lifts. A presence that sharpens and a name that holds weight for generations.

Your Word Is Equity in Every Room

In elite circles, the real currency isn't cash; it's character. Men of power don't waste time verifying credentials when your reputation has already entered the room before you. If your word has weight, the room moves differently. You don't need a pitch deck. You don't need to over-explain. You speak, and they listen because they know you follow through on your promises.

Most men fail when they chase attention, flaunt success, and talk big, but when the pressure hits, they fold, delay, or disappear. Not you. A masculine man doesn't speak unless he's willing to back it with blood, sweat, or signature. That's what makes him rare and respected.

You become the man people call when everything's on the line. Not because you're the cheapest, the flashiest, or the most liked, but because you always deliver. You keep your name clean. You don't promise what you can't deliver, and when you commit, you follow through, even if it costs you.

That's why your word becomes equity. It buys trust. It accelerates deals. It attracts allies. In boardrooms, in negotiations, and high-stakes conversations, your voice doesn't just fill space; it moves decisions because, behind every sentence, there's a solid track record.

Here's the power move most never understand: your legacy becomes the fine print. Contracts will expire. Terms will change, but your word is honoured over the years, becoming the standard others rise to meet.

The Man Who Can Be Trusted Becomes the Man Who Is Followed

When chaos strikes, and emotions run high, people don't follow the loudest voice in the room. They look for the one man who holds the line. The one who doesn't flinch, doesn't chase, doesn't bluff. They look for the man who has already proved, through consistency, that his word is iron.

You're not fighting for attention. You're not performing dominance. You've already shown, over months and years, that when you say you'll show up, you do. That is when the stakes are high, you don't disappear, you deliver. Your word becomes the compass others trust when their vision is clouded.

In the storm, clarity is power. Clarity comes from integrity. The man who keeps his promises, holds his line, and doesn't collapse under pressure becomes the rock around which others build their decisions.

Women feel it. Teams feel it. Investors feel it. They sense that you're not driven by emotion. You don't need permission. You move with quiet certainty and precise action.

May 22nd

When Everything Falls Apart, Integrity Is Your Lifeline

There will be seasons when it all crumbles. The money dries up. Your body gives out. A woman you trusted walks away. The business you built from blood collapses, and in that silence, where men either rise or disappear, you'll face the rawest question a man can ask:

Who am I without it all?

If your identity is all about status, image, or validation, you'll spiral down a hole. If you embody honour, you won't just survive; you'll rebuild with precision.

While others panic, you move, not emotionally, but intentionally. Because you've lived through loss before and never once compromised your core. That's not just resilience. That's unbreakable masculinity.

A man who holds integrity through collapse becomes a dangerous force, not because he's reckless, but because he's grounded. You can take his house, his status, his name, but you can't take his code. That's what allows him to rise faster than those still licking their wounds.

When the dust settles, and people ask, "How did you keep going?" the answer will be simple:

I never lied to myself. I never broke my word. I stayed calm, even when I had nothing to say.

That's how men build empires from ashes.

May 23rd

Trust Is Maintained Under Pressure

Anyone can carry integrity when life is smooth. Absolute trust, the kind that creates undeniable presence, is earned when you're under pressure. When money's tight, pride takes a hit and alone with a decision that no one else will see, that's the test. The man who holds his standard at that moment earns something no follower, faker, or keyboard leader ever will.

When you've walked through what seems like the darkest moments and refused to give up, people feel it without a word spoken. That's authentic masculine leadership, not in what you say but in what you never compromise.

Every next-level masculine man should deliberately put himself in high-risk, high-stakes situations. Not for social media, not for followers, but to meet himself. Do something personal, something no one around you would dare to attempt—a real test for yourself.

Run an ultramarathon with no support and without it being part of an organised event with others. Hike a dangerous peak solo. Swim across a channel.

The key is not to over research it. Don't over plan it. Just commit. Learn by doing. Let it force you into problem-solving, humility, endurance, and raw pride.

That kind of experience forges a level of internal pride that no title or dollar figure can touch. It's the proof that you can rely on yourself. Once you earn that, you carry yourself differently. You walk into a room, and it adjusts. People feel your weight without knowing why.

Action:

1. Choose a personal challenge that scares you, something outside your domain, off the beaten path, with no blueprint.
2. Set a date. No delays. Do it on that date, regardless of the conditions or other events in your life.
3. Commit to doing it solo. No audience. No "content." Just pressure and presence.

You're Only as Powerful as Your Inner Alignment

The world will judge you by your results, your body, your wealth, and your actions. The universe measures you by your alignment. It knows when your actions match your word, when your energy is clean and when your soul isn't at war with your ambition.

You can't hide from that.

A man may build empires, seduce women, and dominate rooms, but if he's fragmented inside, none of it lasts. Sooner or later, the cracks show. The deals fall through. The relationships collapse. Not because he lacked talent but because his spirit wasn't whole.

Masculine strength isn't just physical or mental; it's a matter of spiritual clarity and integrity. It's knowing that who you are in silence, in solitude, in stillness, is the same man the world sees in motion. That kind of integrity doesn't just earn respect; it earns divine momentum. Life starts opening for you. Doors move before you knock. People trust what they feel in your presence, not just what they hear from your mouth.

When you build from that inner stillness, that sacred code, your power stops being performative and starts being magnetic.

Action:

1. Sit in silence today. No phone, no input.
2. Ask yourself: Where am I out of alignment with the man I claim to be?
3. Close your eyes, breathe deep, and promise this: I will move as a masculine man in every space.
4. Follow through. Quietly. Relentlessly.

The Man Who Faces Himself Daily Becomes Untouchable

The masculine man doesn't flinch from hard truths. He doesn't numb out, hide behind success, or distract himself with noise. You sit in the discomfort, your guilt, your failures, the consequences of your choices, and own it all.

That's where the real power is, not in perfection but in full accountability.

You don't get stronger by avoiding yourself; you get stronger by facing yourself head-on each day, stripping the ego, excuses, and denial, and walking out clearer and more grounded. Not for others. For you. A man who trusts himself after facing his darkest moments doesn't need to prove anything. He becomes untouchable.

Self-trust is the armour no one can take away. When everything else goes, money, image, comfort, and relationships are what keep you standing.

Action:

1. Identify the one truth you've been avoiding, a regret, mistake, or fear you haven't faced.

2. Tonight, sit with it. No distraction. No escape. Just own it.

3. Write down what it taught you and how you'll move sharply because of it.

Gratitude Makes Strength Noble

Strength by itself can dominate. It can impress. It can conquer. Without trust and Honour, it turns into ego and performance, and without gratitude, it becomes empty power.

When a man builds his strength on a foundation of earned trust in himself and from others and layers that with genuine gratitude, he transcends, he's no longer proving. He's serving and no longer chasing validation. He's building an impact.

You don't access a deep sense of gratitude without first mastering trust. You can't be grateful for your journey if you've lied your way through it. You can't appreciate your scars if you've hidden them from view. And you can't lead others with gratitude if you don't fully respect the man staring back at you.

Gratitude makes your strength noble. It refines your edge. It humbles your power. It makes people want to follow, not just admire you.

That's where legacy begins, not just in how strong you became but in how honourably you carried that strength and how grateful you were to bear the weight.

Action:

1. Tonight, write down three moments you survived that forged your strength.
2. Next to each, write how it made you better, not just harder.
3. Gratitude isn't softness. It's the stamp on true power.
4. When you master trust, gratitude roots itself deep. That's when your strength becomes unforgettable.

Your Greatest Asset Is Who You Are When No One's Watching

It's easy to perform masculinity. To dress sharp, speak well, lift heavy, and post polished highlights, but none of that builds a legacy. The objective measure of a man, especially at the highest levels, is who he is in silence.

It's how you speak about someone when they're not in the room. It's how you treat the cleaner, not the CEO. It's whether you follow through on your word, even when no one's checking. It's what you do with your phone down, your head clear, and your ego out of the way.

That version of you, the one that never gets posted, is the one people feel. In high-level rooms, in authentic relationships, and in times of pressure, your reputation shows up before your words do. The deeper your character runs behind closed doors, the more power your presence carries everywhere else.

Men who dominate long-term don't need to prove anything externally because they've already earned their respect privately.

Without Honour, Even Strength Turns Against You

Strength without Honour is a loaded weapon with no aim. You might be powerful physically, financially, or intellectually, but without a code to guide that power, you eventually turn it inward or against the people around you.

We've seen it before. Men who look the part. Built bodies. Sharp minds. High-level careers. But no internal compass. They sabotage relationships, burn down partnerships, or collapse under the weight of their ego. Power without Honour is unstable.

Honour is what gives strength its purpose. It's what makes people feel safe under your leadership, not controlled. It's what keeps you grounded when praise is high and steady when storms hit. It's what turns raw power into refined presence.

A man with Honour doesn't need to dominate through fear; he influences through integrity. His strength elevates everything it touches.

Action:

1. Audit your strength today.
2. Where are you using it to serve, and where are you letting it drift toward control or ego?
3. Channel your edge through Honour. That's how you become a force people trust, not just fear.

May 29th

Gratitude Sharpens Perspective, Honour Directs It

Gratitude keeps your feet on the ground, no matter how high you climb. It reminds you where you came from, what you've endured, and who helped you rise. It sharpens your vision because you're not focused on what you lack; you're clear on what truly matters.

Gratitude alone isn't enough. Without Honour, it becomes passive. Sentimental. Lacking edge.

Honour gives that gratitude direction. It's the code that tells you what to protect, what to build, and what to walk away from. It keeps you steady when the ego wants to flex. It holds the line when temptation tries to blur it. Together, gratitude and Honour form the compass of a masculine man with a clear focus.

Stop chasing status. You move with purpose. Stop reacting. You lead. Stop trying to impress. You build an impact that lasts.

May 30th

The Most Respected Man Isn't the Loudest, He's the Clearest

Clarity is power. It's knowing exactly who you are, what you stand for, what you will and won't do, and what your presence represents when you walk into the room—no mixed signals. No overcompensation. Just truth in motion.

The clear man doesn't need to dominate the conversation because everyone's already watching how you move. Your reputation comes through consistency. The way you follow through. The way you honour your word. The way you don't shift to please.

You don't need to chase rooms; rooms talk about you.

You don't fake confidence; you earn it through alignment.

You don't need followers; you lead by being a fixed point in a chaotic world.

That's the masculine man people remember. That's the one they respect when it counts.

When Strength, Trust, Honour, and Gratitude Align, You Become Untouchable

Strength without trust is a threat. Trust without Honour is fragile. Honour without gratitude becomes rigid. When all four live in the same man, you create an unshakeable presence.

You're not just strong — you're reliable.

You're not just reliable — you're principled.

You're not just principled — you're grateful for every test that built you.

That's the edge.

You're the man who can carry weight, not just in the gym but in the boardroom, the relationship, and the battlefield of life. You're trusted because you mean what you say. You're honoured because you do what you say. And you're respected because you appreciate the path, not just the payoff.

It's not one trait. It's the integration.

Action:
Audit yourself across all four: Write one sentence for each. Keep it sharp. Then act on the weakest one today.

1. Strength: Are you physically and mentally training at the level you expect from yourself?
2. Trust: Where are you out of alignment with your word?
3. Honour: What do you know is right that you've been avoiding?
4. Gratitude: Have you given thanks for the pain that has forged you?

June

Gratitude & Abundance

The Warrior's Vision for Expansion

You've survived. You've built. You've endured. Now, it's time to see differently. This month is about unlocking the warrior's lens, where gratitude isn't weakness, and abundance isn't fantasy. It's about recognising everything you've earned, everything you're standing on, and using it as fuel for what's next.

Gratitude isn't about sitting still. It's about becoming aware of your power and then multiplying it. The modern masculine man doesn't whine about what's missing. You extract value from every loss, turn pain into data, and see expansion where others see obstacles.

You don't attract abundance by hoping; you do it by owning and recognising your inner wealth, your discipline, and your path. You become magnetic when you stop chasing and start commanding.

This month, you'll learn to appreciate like a weapon, not a wish. You'll see through the noise and recalibrate your focus to opportunity, alignment, and growth. Gratitude sharpens your awareness. Abundance follows your standard.

The man who truly appreciates what he has moved with such clarity and confidence the world starts giving him more.

"Gratitude sharpens your edge. A man who sees the good sees the way forward."

June 1st

Gratitude Grounds You

Without gratitude, a man's strength can easily mutate into unchecked aggression, action without depth, and force without direction. You might move fast, speak loudly, train hard, and chase power, but if you're doing it all from a place of lack, you're just reacting to life, not leading it.

Gratitude shifts the frequency. It slows the mind, sharpens the senses, and reminds you of what you've already achieved. It puts you back in your body, back in your breath, and back in control. You stop trying to dominate everything and start commanding your lane. That's the difference between being intimidating and being impactful.

A masculine man who's grounded in gratitude doesn't flinch under pressure because he's not trying to prove anything. He's operating from solid ground. He's already won battles that no one saw. He's thankful for the pain that built his edge. That roundedness creates an internal gravity that others feel, especially women. It's safe. It's attractive. It's real.

Gratitude isn't soft; it's stabilising. It holds your power in place, so it doesn't spill recklessly. When everything's loud and chaotic, the grateful man stays calm, collected, and dialled in. That's why people trust him. That's why his strength lasts.

June 2nd

Shift From Scarcity to Strength

Masculine men don't operate from what's missing. Scarcity thinking is reactive, anxious, and weak. It creates a man who grabs, who competes out of fear, who constantly second-guesses his worth. When you shift into gratitude, you activate strength. You recognise that even if you don't have everything you want yet, you've got the passion to earn it.

That shift alters your posture, tone, and decisions. Instead of chasing approval or possessions to fill a void, you lead with presence. That's a masculine energy characterised by stability, expansion, and self-sufficiency.

Action:

1. Write down three things you've built, physically, mentally, or emotionally. Not dreams. Not goals. Wins you've earned.

2. Read them out loud. Breathe them in. Then ask: "What's the next level I can build from this strength, not from lack?"

June 3rd

Recognise the Hidden Wins

Most men look at failure and only see the loss, the missed deal, the breakup, the injury, the setback. A masculine man trains his eyes to see deeper. Every fall, you were taught something. Every time you got back up, you gained a sharper edge. Failure isn't just pain; it's pattern recognition. It's where the power of your purpose is carved, where your threshold is extended, and where your ego is dismantled so the real you can emerge.

Gratitude is what lets you extract the gold. When you stop resenting your past and start mining it, you find the tools forged in fire, sharper judgment, deeper patience, and transcend resilience. That's how you grow from pain, not get buried by it. You don't glorify failure; you respect it. Without it, you'd be soft. Naive. Unproven.

Masculine power is shaped not by perfect wins but by brutal lessons that you turn into leverage.

Action:

1. Pick one of your biggest failures.
2. Write out three things it taught you that made you sharper, stronger, or brighter.
3. Remind yourself: That wasn't a loss. That was my power lesson.

June 4th

You Become a Calm Force

A masculine man grounded in abundance doesn't react; you respond. You don't let the moment control you because you've already positioned yourself with clarity, confidence, and purpose. While others scramble, overthink, or lash out, you remain composed. That calm isn't weakness; it's earned control.

Abundance means you trust yourself. You trust your ability to adapt, to lead, and to rebuild if needed. That internal assurance makes you magnetic. Other men trust you because you're not driven by fear or desperation. Women are drawn to you because your calm signals safety and strength, the kind that doesn't need to flex.

You don't chase, you don't beg, and you never shrink—your position. You lead. You hold. You're not just present; you're grounded, and in today's chaotic world, that's the rarest power a man can carry.

June 5th

Own Your Past Without Bitterness

Masculine power doesn't come from a perfect past; it comes from owning every chapter. The pain, the betrayal, the failures, the choices you wish you'd made differently. A weak man resents the story. A masculine man rewrites the meaning. Every scar has a purpose. Every mistake sharpened him. He doesn't carry shame; he carries structure.

Bitterness is a signal you haven't claimed the lesson. Gratitude clears that out. It turns regret into wisdom and transforms wounds into a source of strength. When you stop trying to erase your past and start honouring it, you stop leaking energy and start walking with real presence.

Action:

1. Write down one part of your past you still resent.
2. Now flip the lens: what strength did it give you? What edge, awareness, or boundary did it build?
   Say it out loud: "This didn't break me. It built me."
3. Move forward like it's true because it is.

June 6th

Start Each Day Grounded, Not Hungry

The masculine man doesn't wake up in reaction mode, checking messages, chasing validation, or reaching for dopamine. He wakes up grounded, clear, present, grateful for the position you've built and prepared to expand it. That shift in energy sets the tone because hunger from lack is noisy, and hunger from purpose is precise.

Gratitude at the start of the day calms the nervous system, sharpens awareness, and puts you back in control. You're not desperate to prove; you're ready to execute. That's the edge. A man who leads his day from a grounded presence walks differently, speaks differently, and moves with command instead of chaos.

Action:

1. Wake up and sit in silence for 3 minutes. No phone. No noise. Just presence.
2. Write down three things you're grateful for and one reason why. Don't rush it.
3. Read your mission aloud. The one-line reason you do what you do.
4. Move your body. Even for 5 minutes. Remind your system who's in control.

June 7th

Refine Your Dominance

Absolute masculine dominance isn't about overpowering; it's about elevating. Weak men try to take space. Masculine men own theirs, then raise the standard for everyone who steps into it. You don't need to bark, beg, or flex. Your energy speaks before your words. Your presence shifts the atmosphere, and the people in it rise, or they leave.

Gratitude is what polishes that dominance. It strips away arrogance and anchors you in purpose. You're not trying to prove anything. You're showing what already is. That's the refinement, power with precision, intensity with intention. When you operate from that place, women feel safe and challenged. Men feel inspired and challenged. You lead without forcing, and that's what makes it respected.

June 8th

See the Pattern in the Pain

When you keep hitting the same wall in life, it's not bad luck; it's a blind spot. Pain isn't random. It's a mirror. It reflects where you haven't paid attention, where you've avoided growth, or where your ego still drives the wheel.

When you stop resenting the pain and start studying it, you step into power. Gratitude allows you to extract the truth, not just the hurt. You begin to see the cycles: in business, in love, and in how you show up. Once you spot the pattern, you can break it. You stop repeating and start rising. That's when pain becomes a tool, not a trap.

You're not here to repeat. You're here to evolve. Masculine men outgrow their patterns and lead with the lessons they have learned.

Action:

1. Write down the last three significant challenges or setbacks you've faced.
2. Under each, list the common denominator: a belief, a behaviour, a reaction.
3. Circle the one that shows up the most; that's you

June 9th

Women Crave Safety and Depth

What truly ignites a woman isn't loud dominance or surface-level bravado. It's presence—a man fully in the moment. A man who listens with his eyes, speaks with clarity, and stands like he's unshaken. That's what makes her nervous system relax and her attraction intensify.

Gratitude is the root of that presence. When you're thankful, not entitled, you slow down. You become aware. You stop grasping and start embodying. That's the energy women trust and desire. It says, 'You're not distracted.' You're here. You're solid.

When she feels that, she opens up emotionally, physically, and energetically. Safety is the doorway to surrender, and depth is the current that keeps her coming back. You don't need to be perfect. You need to be grounded, and gratitude makes that possible, but presence makes it undeniable.

Action:

1. When you're with a woman, no phone, no distractions, no glancing around.
2. Look her in the eyes when she speaks. Hold your posture. Listen without rushing.
3. Before the moment ends, say one thing you genuinely appreciate about her presence.

June 10th

Build Stronger Relationships

When a man operates from gratitude, they no longer search for relationships to fill a void. He doesn't need rescuing, validation, or completion because he's already whole. That shift changes everything.

You become intentional with who you bring into your life. You recognise value in others without attaching your worth to them, and that creates a genuine connection, not dependency.

Gratitude makes you see people for who they are, not just what they can give you. It sharpens discernment, deepens patience, and fuels appreciation. You show up with a calm presence instead of an emotional demand. You lead with clarity instead of insecurity. That makes others feel seen, not used.

You attract partners, friends, and allies who share your values and approach. People who challenge you, build with you and hold you to a higher standard. Relationships stop draining you; they expand you.

June 11th

Attract High-Quality Allies

Masculine men in gratitude don't see the world as a battlefield of threats. They see it as a platform of opportunity. When you're grounded in abundance, you don't need to tear others down to rise; you rise with others, and that energy attracts winners.

Strong men recognise other strong men. When they sense that you're not competing for scraps but building from vision, they want in. You become a magnet for allies who challenge you, expand you, and match your pace. That's how tribes form. That's how empires scale, not through ego but alignment.

Gratitude removes envy. Abundance removes scarcity. The man who leads from both becomes the signal others respect, follow, and build beside.

Action:

1. Reach out to one high-value individual in your network, someone who inspires or challenges you.
2. Acknowledge something you respect. Ask how you can collaborate, contribute, or support.
3. Don't pitch. Don't posture. Just build a connection.

June 12th

Become Magnetic in Business

Gratitude isn't soft; it's strategic. In business, energy is everything. People don't just buy products or services; they buy certainty. When a man leads with grounded appreciation, not desperation, his presence becomes magnetic.

Clients trust him because he listens. Teams follow him because he's composed under pressure. Investors back him because he sees an opportunity where others complain. Gratitude sharpens vision and amplifies leadership; it signals a man who can grow without losing control.

You're not chasing deals. You're attracting alignment. Your clarity makes negotiations cleaner. Your appreciation makes loyalty stronger. In every room, your energy says: This man builds things that last, and others want to be part of that.

June 13th

Reflect on the Storms You've Carried Alone

Every man who walks with quiet strength has weathered storms no one saw—the late nights with doubt. The fights no one could help you win—the moments where it was just you, your will, and the mission.

That version of you, the one who held the line when everything begged you to quit, is the reason you're still standing. It's your edge. Your foundation. You don't need applause for it. You don't need to retell it. But you do need to honour it.

Masculine power isn't just forward-facing. It's backward awareness without emotional attachment. Gratitude toward your inner strength deepens your calm, sharpens your trust, and silences the noise. Once you've carried your storm, no man can shake you.

Action:

1. Tonight, sit in silence for 5 minutes.
2. Think back to one storm, the moment when quitting was easy, but you didn't.

3. Write a note to that version of yourself. One line: "I saw you. I'm proud of you. Thank you."

4. Keep it where you see it often because that man built you.

June 14th

Live Grateful, Move Decisive

A grounded, masculine man in gratitude doesn't stall, overthink, or spiral into doubt. His mindset is clear: I've already won before. I'm here to win again.

Gratitude sharpens your lens. It makes you see possibilities where others see problems. When you operate from that energy, your decisions come faster, cleaner, and with more certainty. You don't get stuck trying to avoid risk; you lean in with purpose.

You don't need the stars to align. You align yourself. You trust your preparation. You trust your pattern of survival and success. Gratitude clears the fog, allowing action to strike.

Masculine presence isn't just about power; it's about precision and control. Gratitude strips the noise. What's left is movement with direction.

June 15th

Appreciate Without Attachment

Gratitude isn't clinging. It's clarity. The masculine man appreciates what he has, who he's with, and where he stands without gripping onto any of it out of fear. That's what makes your energy calm, not chaotic. Desirable, not desperate.

When you're thankful and cantered, you radiate self-assurance. You're not chasing outcomes; you're inviting alignment. Women feel that. It tells them you don't need them to feel whole, which, ironically, makes them want to be around you more. Your presence isn't grasping. It's grounded.

You can love deeply without attachment. Lead without control. Appreciate everything while still standing on your own two feet. That's strength. That's presence. That's how a man attracts from abundance, not from lack.

Action:

1. Today, pick one thing or one person you're deeply thankful for.

2. Write a short note or message of appreciation, no agenda, no outcome expected. Just clear, clean gratitude.

3. Let it go. Don't wait for a response. Watch how powerful you feel simply from expressing without needing to.

June 16th

Radiate Trust Without Speaking

A man grounded in gratitude doesn't enter a room trying to earn approval; you already carry approval within yourself. That's the difference. You're not performing for attention. You walk in like a man who's already won battles no one knows about, and that energy commands respect before you open your mouth.

Gratitude makes you calm. It makes you patient. It strips urgency and gives you presence. It's in that presence that people feel something rare: trust. You don't have to tell them you're solid. They feel it. In the way you move and how you pause. How you listen without the need to interrupt or prove.

When a woman encounters this kind of man, her nervous system settles. She can breathe around you. When other men encounter you, they check themselves, not because you flexed, but because you don't need to.

Gratitude makes that possible because when you're thankful, you're stable. When you're stable, you lead without ever needing to speak first.

June 17th

Don't Compare, Channel

A masculine man doesn't waste energy looking sideways. You know that comparison is a thief of peace, focus, and power. The moment you envy another man's body, success, or relationship, you give away your edge.

Gratitude brings it back.

When you're grateful, you stop thinking, "Why not me?" and start thinking, "What's next for me?" You stop watching and start building. Envy turns into energy. Distraction turns into direction.

Powerful men move by channelling everything. Jealousy? Fuel. Rejection? Redirection. Delay? Discipline. Gratitude clears the fog and clears the way for action. You focus on what you're doing.

No masculine man ever became dominant by comparing. You become dominant by executing.

June 18th

Refine Your Language

Masculine power starts in the way you speak, especially when no one else is listening. Your words aren't just noise; they're commands to your nervous system, signals to your subconscious, and anchors to your identity.

Language rooted in lack sounds like:

"I have to go train."

"I should be grateful."

"I'm trying to get better."

That's weak positioning. It places pressure on you and tells your mind you're under obligation and not in control. That's not how a dominant man moves.

Now shift it:

"I get to train."

"I am grateful."

"I choose to improve."

Gratitude lives in ownership. Language is how you express that ownership out loud. A man who speaks with clarity, certainty, and present-moment power makes others lean in, not because he's loud, but because his words have weight.

It's not just what you say, it's how you say it. A composed, concise, grounded tone always carries further than shouting or filler.

Action:

1. For the next 24 hours, catch every time you say, "have to," "should," "need to," or "try."
2. Replace it instantly with: "get to," "choose to," "will," or say nothing until your words hold power.
3. Speak slower, with fewer words but more intent. Every sentence should sound like a decision, not a maybe.

June 19th

Cultivate Long-Term Discipline

Gratitude isn't just about feeling good; it's about fuelling the follow-through. When you're genuinely grateful for your life, your body, and the opportunities it presents, you stop taking them for granted. You stop dipping in and out of effort. You start showing up.

A masculine man doesn't rely on motivation. He runs on his purpose. Gratitude keeps that purpose clear, especially when the work gets repetitive, exhausting, or invisible to others.

Consistency becomes your edge, not because it's exciting but because it's rare. You train, you lead, you protect, you grow, not occasionally, but daily. That kind of discipline creates weight. People, women, teams, and partners start to depend on your stability because they feel it's not conditional.

You're not disciplined because someone's watching. You're disciplined because you remember why it matters. Masculine strength isn't found in hype. It's in those quiet moments where you choose consistency out of gratitude.

Action:

1. Before your next training session, work task, or relationship effort, pause for 30 seconds.

2. Ask yourself: "What do I appreciate about this challenge right now?"

3. Say it out loud, then act, not to check a box, but to honour the opportunity.

June 20th

Women Stay, Not Just Show Up

Masculine dominance might catch her eye, but it's your depth that keeps her close. Anyone can attract. Few can hold.

When you're grounded in gratitude, your energy shifts from proving to providing. You're not chasing approval. You're appreciating presence. Women feel that difference instantly. You're not the kind of person who needs her to validate your worth; you already know who you are.

Gratitude gives your dominance direction. It shows your strength isn't just about control; it's about care. You're powerful but present. Commanding, but grounded. That balance is what makes women feel something more profound than attraction; it makes them feel safe, seen, and wanted for who they are, not just what they give.

Gratitude says: I don't need to own you. I choose to honour you.

Action:

1. Next time you're with a woman, partner, date, or friend, stop scrolling, stop planning, stop performing.
2. Look her in the eyes. Listen fully. Let your energy say, "I'm right here."
3. Say something simple but real: "I appreciate this moment with you."

June 21ˢᵗ

Use Stillness as a Weapon

In a world addicted to noise, speed, and showing off, the masculine man who knows how to be still becomes a rare and commanding presence. Stillness isn't weakness; it's a form of containment. You're grounded

Gratitude feeds that stillness. It quiets the ego that says, "Do more. Prove more. Be more." Instead, it reminds you, "You are already grounded. Now move from alignment, not reaction."

Stillness allows your intuition to surface. You feel what's real. You make better decisions. You spot the lie in the deal, the tension in the room, the truth in the silence. You respond with power, not panic.

To women, this stillness is magnetic. It says you're not desperate. You're deliberate. To men, it isn't very safe, not because you're loud, but because your silence carries weight.

A warrior moves with purpose. Not rushed. Not shaken. Just ready. Stillness is your edge. Gratitude is the blade. Keep it sharp. Use it wisely.

Action:

1. Wake up, sit down, and put your phone away.

2. Breathe slowly. In through your nose. Hold. Out through your mouth.

3. Focus on this one thought: "What am I grateful for right now, and what needs my calm action today?"

June 22nd

Don't Burn Out, Burn Brighter

Gratitude is what keeps the fire lit without letting it consume you. It turns pressure into power, not by pushing harder, but by helping you recognise the value in every demand you face. You're no longer operating from a place of emptiness or ego. It's your drive for purpose, clarity, and self-respect.

Burnout occurs when a person forgets why they started. When you chase status instead of substance. A person grounded in gratitude stays connected to the reason behind their work. You don't give your time to everything, only to what matters.

You protect your energy because you know what it creates: impact, attraction, and legacy, not from grinding 24/7 but from moving with precision. That's why high-level men appear calm while handling pressure; they remain centred.

Women feel this deeply. She sees a man who isn't reactive but intentional. You don't burn out trying to prove; you burn brighter by staying true to your alignment. That's the kind of man who builds empires and families and doesn't collapse under the weight of either.

June 23rd

Attract Wealth Naturally

Wealth doesn't chase noise. It follows clarity. Clarity comes from a man who knows who he is, what he stands for, and what he already has.

Gratitude flips the script. Instead of operating from lack, "I need more, I'm not there yet, I must hustle to be worthy", you move to a place of already having value. You're not proving yourself to money, investors, or opportunity. You invite it through presence, precision, and power.

Gratitude is what makes your energy clean. You're not grasping, begging, or manipulating. You're focused, appreciative, and unshakeable. That's when high-level networks, teams, and deals succeed, not from desperation but disciplined confidence.

When you live in abundance, you see opportunities where others see threats. You recognise the people worth building with. You know when to move, when to pause, when to receive. Real and sustaining wealth flows to that frequency.

Action:

1. Each morning, list three things you already have that signal value: skillsets, relationships, insights, and experiences.

2. Ask: "How can I move today in a way that honours and multiplies these?"
3. Step into conversations, work, and decisions as if you're already wealthy.

Make Wealth a By-product, not a Goal

The masculine man doesn't chase money; he builds value, and wealth follows.

There is a sharp difference between the man obsessed with appearing rich and the man committed to being valuable. One performs. The other produces. One flexes online. The other builds quietly and gets paid loudly.

Abundance moves faster toward the grounded man who leads with presence, power, and clarity. Why? Because people can feel when your outcome-hungry versus mission-driven. When your focus is solely on the payday, your energy becomes desperate. You compromise standards. You bend the truth. You grab whatever's in reach instead of building something that lasts.

When wealth is the result, not the target, your moves get cleaner. You focus on solving real problems, mastering your craft, and staying aligned with your code. That energy is magnetic to high-level rooms, elite networks, clients, investors, and partners. You're not asking for attention. You're earning respect. With it, income, ownership, and equity.

You become the man who brings something rare to the table: stability with strength, clarity with confidence. That's when the money chases you. Not for who you pretend to be but for who you've become.

June 25th

Gratitude Becomes a Force Multiplier

Most men are reactive. Triggered by setbacks, distracted by success, swinging between entitlement and burnout. A man with gratitude doesn't react; you radiate. Your power doesn't come from force; it comes from clarity. From being anchored in what's working and what's real.

Your strength becomes steadier because you're no longer chasing validation; you're building from a solid core. Your clarity sharpens not by envy or self-pity; you're focused on what's actionable. Your trust deepens in yourself and others because people feel your consistency. Your presence is clean.

Gratitude amplifies your leadership. It magnifies your presence in relationships. It scales your impact in business. When your energy is abundant, people lean in. They want to build with you, buy from you, follow you, and open up to you.

When you live with gratitude, you multiply more than just results.

You multiply respect.

You multiply desire.

You multiply legacy.

June 26th

Lead Without Force

You don't need to push. You don't need to be convinced. When your presence is aligned, your decisions are clean, and your energy is stable, people lean in. They trust where you're going because you're not leading for applause. You're leading with direction.

This kind of leadership isn't loud. It's felt. In your eye contact. In your calm under pressure. In the way, you say less but move with intent. You're not selling a vision; you are the vision. That's why others follow. Not out of fear but because they believe in the way you walk.

You don't dominate the room by force; you shift it with focus. That's what real masculine presence does. It creates movement without needing noise—influence without needing attention.

June 27th

The Abundant Man Sees
the Patterns

Masculine men don't just appreciate the wins; they honour the lessons inside the losses.

Every recurring challenge in your life is a message wrapped in repetition. That same tension in your relationship. That friction in business. That emotional dip that shows up every few months. These aren't inconveniences. They're insights, and when gratitude and abundance are intense, you stop resisting them and start receiving them.

Life is always giving you feedback. The abundant man sees it. The masculine man uses it.

You don't say, "Why does this keep happening to me?"

You say, "What pattern is life showing me, and what's the opportunity in it?"

This shift in perspective reframes life from a battleground into a training ground.

Action: (30 Minutes)

1. Write down three areas where friction keeps showing up: emotional triggers, recurring arguments, and delayed outcomes. Nothing is random. These are your keys.

2. Where are you showing up in the same way each time? Is it control? Doubt? Guilt? Get honest. Gratitude means you can face the truth without flinching.

3. Ask: What is this here to teach me? Is it boundaries? Patience? Courage? Leadership? Track it, honour it.

4. Write down one new action, mindset, or response you will take next time this pattern shows up. Lock it in.

You Leave a Legacy of Strength, Not Scar Tissue

The masculine man doesn't just overcome; he integrates. He doesn't carry his pain like armour. He refines it into wisdom. That's the difference between surviving life and mastering it.

Without gratitude, your victories come at the cost of inner erosion. You win the game, but you lose the peace. Your body might be strong, your bank account full, and your name respected, but inside, you're still bleeding from battles you never processed.

Gratitude changes that. It doesn't make you soft. It makes you solid. It turns pain into perspective. It slows you down just enough to reflect, not react. In that stillness, the masculine man evolves.

Strength without reflection creates collateral damage, broken relationships, explosive reactions, and emotional shutdown. That's not power. That's residue.

When you lead with presence, appreciate your path, and recognise how every scar shaped your edge, you don't just lead well; you last long. You stop passing down pain. You start passing down power.

June 29th

Gratitude Anchors Vision in Reality

The high-level masculine man doesn't fantasise about the future; he builds it from a grounded presence. That presence is in gratitude.

Gratitude isn't just about looking back with appreciation; it's about standing firmly in what is while holding the clarity of what will be. Most men get lost chasing an imagined ideal, constantly feeling behind, unfulfilled, and unsatisfied. When you live from abundance, you stop grasping. You start creating.

That's the edge: masculine vision rooted in grounded energy. You don't chase, you channel. You're not trying to escape where you are; you're building upward from it. That's why your progress sticks. That's why your relationships deepen. That's why your leadership lands.

You're not moving from emptiness; you're moving from embodiment.

Gratitude Is the Gateway to Love, Leadership, and Connection

When a man lives from breath, you master presence.

When a man builds his strength, you earn power.

When a man walks in trust, you become unshakable.

When that man adds gratitude, everything expands.

Gratitude is not softness. It's precision. It's how a man tempers his fire, so it warms instead of burns. It's the fuel behind calm confidence, behind clean decisions, behind staying the course when everything else begs for chaos. Gratitude isn't a feeling; it's an operating system. When it runs deep, it turns strength into service, power into presence, and clarity into connection.

The highest masculine frequency isn't noise; it's depth. It's silence that speaks. Breath that calms. A gaze that grounds and a presence that loves, not from need, but from overflow.

A masculine man in full, forged through pressure, refined through discipline, guided by purpose, and elevated by gratitude. The more you see what is, the more you're trusted with what can be.

Love & Relationships

Love Fiercely. Lead with Integrity. Build Bonds Worthy of a Legacy

This month isn't about the game. It's about grounded love, masculine connection, and how to build relationships that don't dilute your mission; they amplify it.

A connection starts with you being real. The kind of man who speaks with clarity, protects without control, and holds a frame even when emotions are high. Masculine love isn't soft; it's fierce, strong, and primal. It holds space while still setting boundaries, and when you master it, you become the man women respect, desire, and trust, not because of charm but because of your consistency.

This month, you'll learn to lead your relationships with integrity, not insecurity. You'll attract from strength, not scarcity. You'll hold your line without shutting down, and you'll begin to understand that real masculine love doesn't take away your power; it refines it.

A man who can protect, provide, and be fully present without ever losing himself is the rarest kind. The kind the world needs more of.

"Masculine love isn't soft; it's steady, protective, and unshakably present."

July 1st

Start With Self-Respect

Before you can lead in love, you need to lead yourself. That starts with how you speak to yourself, how you treat your body, and how you keep your word when no one's watching. If your self-respect is low, your standards will reflect it, and you'll accept behaviour, energy, and relationships that match your inner doubts.

You don't attract what you want. You attract what you allow.

Masculine men do not beg for attention. They choose themselves first through discipline, integrity, and ownership, a frequency that repels drama and magnifies depth.

Boundaries are how you love yourself out loud. You don't overextend. You don't stay where you're disrespected. You don't chase approval. You move from clarity.

When you hold that frame, the right woman doesn't try to break it. She relaxes into it. Your self-respect gives her something to trust.

Action:

1. Where are you tolerating energy that drains you?
2. Where are you shrinking to keep peace or affection?
3. What boundary have you been avoiding enforcing?

July 2nd

Build Emotional Control, Not Suppression

Masculine men don't pretend they don't feel; they refine how they handle their emotions. Suppression is weakness dressed up as calmness. It leaks through passive aggression, outbursts, withdrawal, or addiction. That's not control; that's collapse in slow motion.

Absolute control is mastery. You feel anger, sadness, and pain, but you choose how to respond to them. You breathe through it. You process it. Then, you speak or act with clarity, not chaos.

Masculine men are safe to love, not because they're emotionless but because they're grounded. When a woman sees you experience emotion without losing yourself in it, she trusts you more and feels freer to express herself fully, knowing you won't react like a boy; you'll respond like a man.

Action:

Next time you're emotionally triggered:

1. Breathe. Deep and slow. Create space.
2. Name it. "This is frustration," "This is disappointment."
3. Ask yourself: "What's the real reason I feel this?"
4. Speak with intention or choose silence with strength.

July 3rd

Attract Feminine Energy Naturally

Feminine energy responds to one thing above all: the presence of the masculine. Not performance. Not pretence. Presence. The kind that doesn't flinch when tested. The kind that stays grounded when the world sways. That doesn't need explaining; it only needs to be embodied.

When you walk with deep internal trust, women feel it. In the calmness of your breath. In the directness of your eye contact. In the way, you move without needing applause. A grounded man doesn't force attraction. You radiate it.

She doesn't want a man who overpowers her. She wants a man who is grounded enough to hold her, both emotionally and physically. When she senses you're not looking to her to complete you but to complement you, she softens. She shifts. She responds.

Your steadiness makes her feminine. Your direction makes her safe. Your depth makes her stay.

July 4th

Create Deep Emotional Loyalty

When a woman feels truly safe, not just physically but emotionally and energetically, she relaxes into you, not out of obligation, but out of desire. She stops protecting herself and starts revealing herself. That's when you stop receiving the surface version of her and begin experiencing the full spectrum of her love, her emotions, and her sexuality.

This depth of connection doesn't come from charm. It comes from consistency. From showing up as the same grounded man in every situation, calm in her chaos, firm in your word, and clear in your actions. That's what makes her open, stay, and pour into you thoroughly.

When she knows, she doesn't need to carry the relationship, she'll double her investment in it. You become her chosen space of freedom, exploration, and surrender. She becomes fiercely loyal, not because you asked her to be, but because you made it safe for her to be.

Emotional loyalty isn't luck. It's through presence, consistency, and being the rock, she never has to doubt. That's high-level masculine leadership in love.

Action:

1. Stop reacting, start responding. When a woman is emotional, don't match her energy. Hold it. Breathe. Stay composed.

2. Let your words match your actions over time. There are no mixed signals. No big promises with weak delivery.

3. Create a space where she can express herself without punishment. You don't need to fix everything; listen to her without judgment.

4. Keep your masculine frame in moments of intimacy and challenge. When she sees you handle both with equal strength, she trusts deeper.

July 5th

Lead With Integrity, Not Control

The high-level masculine man understands that leadership in a relationship is not about power plays or emotional manipulation; it's about trust, intention, and clarity. Leading with integrity means you don't need to dominate to be felt. You don't need to silence her voice to hear your own. Your decisions factor in her safety, your actions reflect her heart, and your presence builds and never breaks.

Control comes from insecurity. Integrity comes from grounded confidence. A man who leads with integrity listens deeply, chooses intentionally, and moves with her, not against her. You lead with strength, but it's not the kind that forces obedience. It's the kind that earns respect.

When you lead like this, you don't just make her feel heard; you make her feel valued and supported. In that space, love deepens. She doesn't resist your leadership; she flows with it. Not because she's weaker but because she feels empowered by the direction you bring.

The core of masculine love is a warrior with an open heart. You guide without force. You protect without possession. You serve without sacrifice, and in that alignment, love thrives, and so does she.

July 6th

Your Relationship Becomes a Fortress

When a masculine man stands grounded in his leadership, and his woman trusts enough to rest in her feminine self, the relationship stops leaking energy. You no longer fight each other. You face the world together.

The masculine sets the tone, provides clear direction, fosters emotional steadiness, and maintains an unwavering presence. The feminine responds with openness, intuition, creativity, and depth. When those forces are respected and not reversed, something powerful happens; external chaos doesn't get in.

Others argue. You adapt. Others break down. You breathe through the storms, and the foundation holds. No drama, ego, or control. Grounded in truth, mutual respect, and roles that empower both.

You become untouchable, not because you avoid struggle, but because of your calm inner strength, and her softness amplifies your strength. Your strength protects her softness. That's not a weakness. That's the highest level of love.

A relationship like this doesn't just survive; it becomes a part of your power and legacy.

July 7th

Learn Her Nervous System

Masculine men don't guess; they study. If you genuinely want to lead with love, you need to understand the woman in front of you at a nervous system level, not as a mystery to be decoded, but as a dynamic being who feels everything more deeply than she can express.

Women are nervous system-based creatures. Safety, arousal, trust, and surrender don't come from words; they come from how you make her feel in her body. If she's tense, she won't open up. If she's anxious, she won't trust you. If she's grounded around you, she'll show you the deepest parts of herself, emotionally and physically and open up to you like no one else.

Action: (Do This Weekly)

1. Observe Without Reacting: The next time she's activated, upset, anxious, or overwhelmed, refrain from trying to fix her. Watch. Breathe slower. Speak slower. Match her with grounded stillness. Let her storm pass with you, not at you.

2. Ask Without Ego: When she's calm, ask, "When do you feel most safe with me?"

   "When do you feel most drawn to me?" "When do you feel misunderstood?"

3. Track Her Cues: Notice her breath, voice, and eyes. Learn her cues. Does she shut down when you interrupt? Open up when you stay silent? Her nervous system is talking. Are you listening?

4. Regulate Yourself First: Your emotional tone is her thermostat. If you can't stay grounded, she won't feel safe. Meditate. Train. Breathe. Master your system before trying to lead hers.

July 8th

Know Your Archetype

Your relationship doesn't start with her; it begins with how you show up. Masculine men don't guess who they are; they know. In love, that self-awareness distinguishes the men who build devotion from those who destroy it.

Each archetype brings a pattern. Some lead. Some follow—some sabotage. The man who studies his wiring, refines it, and chooses growth becomes the partner she trusts, desires, and stays with.

1. Alpha: Driven, dominant, outspoken. Alphas lead from the front. They're confident, assertive, and naturally command attention.

   They make decisions fast. Take control of rooms. However, when immature, they can become arrogant, aggressive, and overly validation hungry.

   Refined Alpha: Calm, grounded, responsible for others. It doesn't need to be proven — only improved. Presence speaks louder than volume.

2. Beta: Reliable, loyal, agreeable. Betas value harmony and avoid conflict. They're often emotionally intelligent but fear rejection.

   In relationships, they can be dependable but may become passive, over-accommodating, or overly available.

Refined Beta: Maintains empathy while adding backbone. Speaks truth without shrinking. He still serves, but from strength, not submission.

3. Gamma: Smart but resentful. Gammas hide behind intellect, sarcasm, or passive aggression. They feel overlooked by the Alphas and envy the attention they receive.

   They often feel like the world owes them, and relationships become emotional landmines.

   Refined Gamma: Converts insight into ownership. Trades jealousy for the journey. He builds himself into someone admired, not just understood.

4. Sigma: Independent, observant, unbothered. Sigmas don't chase the hierarchy; they opt out of it. Mysterious and self-reliant.

   Unchecked, they become isolated, emotionally unavailable, and self-centred in their relationships.

   Refined Sigma: Moves with silent power but knows when to open. He leads himself and makes space for others to rise, too.

5. Zeta: Anti-authority. Nonconformist. Zetas reject structure, roles, and systems. They follow their code, often brilliant but misunderstood.

   Their downfall? Bitterness. Rebellion becomes an identity. They fight everything, even their evolution.

   Refined Zeta: Builds his kingdom with discipline, not just defiance. He makes peace with the structure he creates. He doesn't just rebel; he refines.

6. Delta: Hardworking. Overlooked. Deltas often carry weight but lack direction. They do what's asked but rarely rise to what's possible.

They avoid risk, fear attention, and stay stuck in quiet resentment.

Refined Delta: Wakes up. Finds fire. Turns routine into ritual and starts moving with a mission, not just motion.

7. Omega: Detached, nihilistic, and often self-destructive. Omegas have usually given up on the game; they feel they don't belong and don't care.

But under the cynicism is usually a pain — abandonment, failure, rejection.

Refined Omega: Reconnects to purpose. Learns discipline. Rebuilds not for attention but redemption. He chooses to lead himself out of the shadow into clarity.

Masculine progression is knowing where you are, refining what you carry, and walking daily toward the man who commands life through presence, strength, trust, gratitude, love, and connection.

July 9th

Balance Her, Lead Yourself

A masculine man doesn't fear the feminine; he learns to understand it, and that's the evolution most men avoid. They master dominance, success, and direction but remain emotionally one-dimensional. That's why their relationships plateau; intimacy feels confusing, and she doesn't fully open up because you're not yet safe enough for her to express herself fully.

Learning about feminine and masculine energy isn't about being soft; it's about being strategic.

Yin and Yang. Black and white.

One receives. One initiates.

One feels. One focuses.

They're not opposites. They're partners.

Yin is her, the feminine current. It moves downwards, inward, fluid like the moon. Intuition. Sensitivity. Emotion. She feels everything. She expands in stillness, surrenders in safety, and expresses what the world teaches us to suppress.

Yang is you, the masculine edge. It moves upwards and outward, structured like the sun. Logic. Direction. Determination. You are the container. The rock. The fire she wants to dance around, not be burned by.

When these energies are misaligned in a man, relationships collapse:

- Too masculine, you become controlling, reactive, or emotionally unavailable.
- Too feminine, you become avoidant, passive, over-sensitive, or indecisive.

The woman in your life doesn't just want a provider; she wants a partner. She wants a man who can see her, feel her, and lead her without dimming her flame. When she feels you've studied her nervous system, not just her body, she begins to relax. She blooms. She trusts.

In return, you get her devotion, her desire, and her depth.

Masculine mastery in love begins when you step out of self-interest and into awareness.

July 10th

Lead Her Without Words

A masculine man doesn't wait for her to break down to notice. He senses the shift before the words ever leave her lips. When her vibration changes, when her eyes dim slightly, her body tenses, or her tone shortens, that's your cue. Not to fix. Not to force. But to feel.

You guide her back to softness without speaking a word. No announcements. No "what's wrong?" interrogations. No power plays. Just calibrated, conscious redirection of energy, led through masculine awareness.

Action:

1. Feel the Frequency Before the Feedback: You must be fully tuned in. If the woman's tone sharpens, shoulders rise, and breath shortens, it's likely that emotional energy is building in her nervous system. Don't respond with logic. Respond with leadership.

2. Break the Pattern Subtly: Change the music. Pull her into your arms without asking. Adjust the lighting. Light a candle. Offer her tea or chocolate. Let your body say, "I've got you."

3. Move Her Energy, Not Her Emotions: Guide her gently into a state of flow. Put on a rhythm that pulls her hips

back into movement. Grab her hand. Dance slowly in the kitchen. Keep it quiet. Grounded. Present. You're not solving; you're dissolving.

4. Channel Her Emotion With Your Stability: If she needs a space to release her emotions, offer one. Lead her into movement, into breath, into body. Not dramatic. Just seamless transitions. You hold the storm, and she lets go.

5. Don't Seek Credit. Stay Present.: She will know what you're doing, and she will appreciate it more because you don't need applause for it. You just led. That's what calms her nervous system. That's what earns her trust.

July 11th

Drop the Ego, Keep the Edge

A masculine man in love doesn't use his power to dominate the relationship; instead, he uses it to deepen it. You don't posture, you don't play games, and you don't need to prove anything. Your presence already says it all.

The ego is often a mask for insecurity. It's the need to be right, to control, to protect pride over partnership. When you bring ego into a relationship, you start treating your woman like an opponent, not an ally.

Keeping your edge means staying grounded in who you are without having to crush her spirit to feel strong. You don't shrink back, but you don't overshadow. You speak clearly, but you listen deeply. You lead with direction, but never forget to lead with care.

When a man drops his ego but keeps his edge, his relationship becomes a sanctuary, not a battlefield. She doesn't have to walk on eggshells. She knows your fire won't burn her; it warms her. When things get tense, she doesn't brace for war; she leans in, knowing your strength isn't explosive; it's grounding.

You become the man she trusts not just with her body but with her truth, and that's when love becomes unshakable.

July 12th

Give Without Keeping Score

The masculine man doesn't tally favours. You don't hold his effort hostage. You give not to earn validation but to anchor the connection. Your presence is a gift. Your consistency is the investment. Your love doesn't come with strings attached; it comes with strength.

Keeping score is transactional. It's the insecure attempt to manage love through control, and that's not leadership; that's leverage. Real masculine energy leads with depth, not deals.

You give not to gain but because it's who you are. You listen fully, not because you're waiting your turn to speak, but because her expression matters. You provide stability, not because it wins points, but because chaos dies in your presence. You show up again and again without reminding her what you've done.

That level of devotion multiplies respect and desire. Your woman leans in, not because she's indebted, but because she feels deeply valued. Gratitude grows. Loyalty strengthens. Intimacy deepens.

July 13th

Become a Model for Other Men

How you treat your woman isn't just about your relationship; it's about her. It's a live example of what strength with heart looks like. Other men are always watching: your friends, your peers, your future sons, whether you realise it or not, you're giving them a blueprint.

A masculine man doesn't perform his love. He embodies it. He doesn't belittle her in public. He doesn't flex dominance to appear strong. He leads with integrity, steady, grounded, and unwavering, and when she glows in your presence, the message becomes clear:

"This is how it's done."

It sets a new standard not just for relationships but for manhood.

Real masculine love is rare, not because it's hard to feel, but because it's hard to hold with power. Be the example. Be the edge. Be the man other men silently admire, not for your words, but for the strength of how you love.

Action:
Spend one day intentionally observing how you show up for your woman in front of others:

1. Do you cut her off or invite her voice?
2. Do you lead decisions or control them?
3. Do you create safety in conversation or tension?
4. Does your body language reflect protection or distraction?

Protect Her Energy Like Your Own

A masculine man doesn't just protect his woman physically; he protects her energetically. That means shielding her from chaos, not adding to it. It means choosing clarity over confusion and direction over disorder. When a woman feels emotionally safe, she opens up. When she feels energetically drained by you, she shuts down slowly and then all at once.

It's in the way you look at her, not distracted, not darting around the room, but locked in. Focused. Like she's the only one there. That kind of eye contact settles her nervous system. It says, "You're safe. I'm here. I've got this."

It's in the way you lead decisions, not for her, but with her in mind. You create space for her softness to flourish. You move in ways that preserve her emotional clarity, especially when the world is heavy on her shoulders.

It's in the way you protect time together, with no scrolling and no zoning out. Undivided attention becomes an act of leadership. She reads everything: your tone, your posture, your focus. If you're distracted, she carries more. If you're grounded, she melts.

When she's your queen, you don't add noise to her system. You help her return to herself.

That's how you lead in love, with discipline, with depth, and with energetic precision. A woman's energy is sacred, and a man who truly values her doesn't just protect her body; he shields her peace, and from that place, she gives him the deepest parts of herself.

July 15th

Sex Becomes Deeper,
Not Just Hotter

When a man lives in a full masculine embodiment, grounded in presence, anchored in discipline, and aligned in purpose, sex stops being a performance and becomes an expression.

The feminine craves depth, not just intensity and most men miss this.

You don't chase heat without creating safety. You don't go hard without first going deep. True masculine energy doesn't just arouse; it awakens. It opens her. It reveals her. It allows her to surrender in ways even she hasn't felt before.

This kind of sex commands connection, breath-to-breath, skin-to-skin, energy-to-energy. It starts with how you carry yourself throughout the day. In how you look at her across the room. How you listen, and how you lead decisions with clarity. Your strength, your stillness, your self-control, it all builds anticipation.

When the moment comes, she doesn't just feel your touch; she feels your intention. Your respect. Your hunger. Your restraint. Your presence.

She lets go entirely, not because of technique, but because she trusts you.

This kind of sex is rare. It's spiritual, primal, and deeply human all at once. Her nervous system calms. Her pleasure expands. Time slows down, and she remembers this moment, not for how wild it was, but for how whole it made her feel.

What the Masculine Man Can Do Tonight to Make Her Feel Fully Loved

You don't need to be a tantric master. You don't need years of training. What she truly wants is all of you, your depth, your attention, your certainty, poured into her, without distraction, without ego, and without a clock ticking in your mind.

Action: (tonight)

1. Set the tone, not the schedule: Dim the lights. Light a few candles, not for show, but to create an atmosphere that says, I prepared this for you.

2. Play soft, slow music, not for background noise, but to pace your energy. Let the room feel like a sanctuary. Safe. Intimate. Free from the world.

3. Give her your hands without rushing: Run her a warm bath if you want to start soft. Dry her slowly. Lay her down. Then, start with a massage that is not mechanical, not goal driven. Just focus on her entirely. One hand on her skin. One hand grounds her heart. Breathe slowly. Let her feel your calm.

4. Bring sweetness to her senses: Place one piece of high-quality chocolate between her lips slowly. Let her taste it while you hold her gaze. You're not feeding her food. You're feeding her devotion. That one simple act, done with love, says more than a thousand compliments.

5. Give her one perfect rose, and don't hand it to her: Run it slowly along her body. Over her collarbone. Her stomach. The inside of her thighs. Not to tease but to honour. You're not rushing toward the main event. She is the event.

6. Say less. Breathe more deeply: Your voice should be calm, clear, and confident. Don't overtalk. Let your silence be comfort, not distance. Let your breath sync with hers. When she opens her eyes and sees you grounded, still, and undistracted, she feels a sense of safety. That's what opens her deeper than any line ever could.

7. Give her your whole body, not just your touch: Lean in with intention. Move with purpose. Don't perform, connect. Kiss slowly. Hold her firmly. Stay completely present. No phone. No TV. No wandering minds. Just her. Just now. Let your energy say, I'm' here.' With all of me. For all of you.

8. When it's over, don't roll away. Hold her. Stroke her hair. Kiss her shoulder. Let her know she is worshipped, not used. Masculine love isn't about what you get. It's about what you give from the depths of your stillness, your strength, and your presence. Tonight, give her all of you.

Clear With Your Words, Calm with Your Movements

If she's your queen, her peace becomes your responsibility, not as a possession, but as a sacred partnership.

The high-level masculine man understands that a woman's nervous system is susceptible to her environment, and you are her environment. Your tone, your presence, your decisions, your chaos, or calm, she feels it all, not in words, but in energy.

To protect her energy is to be conscious of how your leadership impacts her flow.

If you're disorganised, she becomes anxious.

If you're inconsistent, she becomes ungrounded.

If you're emotionally erratic, she becomes hypervigilant.

If you're so self-focused that you stop tuning into her, she quietly burns out while trying to hold the space you should have secured.

When you're clear in your words, calm in your movements, sharp in your direction, and firm in your values, she relaxes. Her body opens. Her feminine essence flows. Not because she's weak. It's because your grounded masculine presence makes her feel safe to be her whole self.

Protecting her energy means you handle yours first. You lead with clarity, so she doesn't have to question. You show up consistently so she can settle into a rhythm. You keep drama out of the relationship, just as you would defend your home from a threat. To a woman, emotional chaos is a threat.

Elevating her means considering her well-being in your decisions. It means setting boundaries with people or environments that drain her. It means noticing when she's overloaded and not adding to the fire but being the water that calms it.

Masculine men don't exhaust their women. They regulate themselves so she doesn't have to.

In return, she brings softness, radiance, and trust that most men never get to witness because most men never earned the right to protect her peace in the first place.

July 18th

Train for Depth, Not Just Desire

Any man can spark a moment of desire. The masculine man who understands true love and partnership doesn't just chase heat; he cultivates depth because while desire gets her attention, only depth keeps her devotion.

Depth is presence. It's the way you look at her without distraction. It's the way your silence says more than your compliments. It's the strength in your stillness, not the force in your words. It's the consistency in your actions, even when no one is watching.

Desire fades when it's not grounded. Depth is what she remembers when she's alone. It's what anchors her during her storms. It's the space you create where her soul feels safe to land, not just her body.

Masculine depth is evident in how you ask her how she truly is and then listen. It shows in how you hold her with patience, not possession, in how you don't flinch when she shows all of her: wild, soft, scared, sensual. you've trained for it. You've sat in your discomfort. You've studied the language of your own emotions. You've earned clarity through chaos, and now, you hold her through hers.

July 19th

Eliminate Performance Anxiety

Performance anxiety lives in the head. Presence lives in the body. When a man tries to "perform," he disconnects from himself, from her, from the moment. When you lead from presence, not pressure, intimacy becomes effortless. It's not about technique. It's about connection.

She doesn't want a performance.
She wants you to be grounded, attentive, and connected.
She wants to feel your breath, not your tension.
She wants to experience your depth, not your doubt.

When you stop trying to impress her and start being with her, everything changes. The pressure fades. The flow begins. You move in sync. You feel more.

Action:

1. Breathe Before You Touch: Step back. Inhale deep through your nose for seven seconds, hold for two, and exhale for seven. Do it five times. Calm your nervous system—Anchor in your body. Let your energy drop from your head into your chest.

2. Eye Contact, No Words: Before anything physical, stand close to each other. Look into her eyes without talking for 60 seconds. Let the silence build tension, not awkwardness. That eye contact tells her you're here, fully. It invites her in. She'll feel it.

3. Set Intention, Not Expectation: Silently say to yourself, "I'm here to connect, not to prove."

July 20th

She Stays Because You're Still Growing

She didn't fall for you just because you were strong, sharp, or grounded. She fell for who you were becoming. That edge. That hunger. That refusal to remain the same person, year after year.

A woman grounded in her feminine wants moves toward growth, not chaos. She doesn't crave a finished product. She desires a man committed to your evolution—one who keeps sharpening, expanding, and deepening for yourself, not just for her.

As you continue to grow, you continue to lead. Not with pressure but with presence. Not by dominating but by elevating. She watches you expand and feels safer. More turned on. Prouder because you're not just the man she said yes to; you're the man she'd say yes to again. Not because you're perfect, but because you're becoming.

July 21st

Become Her Safe Space

The masculine man doesn't just stand firm when things are easy; he stays anchored when emotions rise when life hits hard, and when the moment gets messy. That's when she truly feels it: this is her place to fall apart and be held, not fixed.

She doesn't need a solution; she needs your stillness. Your breath slows hers. Your presence regulates her nervous system. Your eyes remind her: "You're safe here. All of you."

Action:

1. Turn off your phone. No distractions.
2. Sit beside her, eye to eye.
3. Ask, "How are you feeling tonight?" Then listen. No advice. No fixing.
4. Place your hand on her lower back or heart and breathe slowly. Match her rhythm.
5. When she finishes speaking, hold the silence. Let her feel seen, not rushed.

July 22nd

Strength She Can Feel

As a high-level masculine man, you don't train just for yourself; you train with your woman in mind. Every hard rep, cold plunge, and mission isn't just about your body or business; it's about building the capacity to lead and protect. Your woman doesn't need soft promises; she wants to feel your depth in how you carry pressure, stay calm under fire, and never let the outside chaos bleed into her world.

Strength in the gym means nothing if you crumble at home. Depth is built in silence, through discipline, through purpose, through how you move when no one's watching. You don't train for applause. You train because she deserves a man who walks in with peace, power, and presence.

Action:

1. Train today with her in mind.
2. Follow through with one action she didn't ask for, done entirely, quietly, like a king.
3. Let your discipline speak the love words you don't have to say.

July 23rd

Be Relentlessly Honest

Lies, even small ones, corrode the core of intimacy. They break more than trust; they break safety. Once safety is gone, the connection fades, regardless of how intense the attraction may be.

Masculine love doesn't hide. It doesn't bend the truth to avoid discomfort. It faces the moment with a backbone. If you've failed, say it. If you're off-track, own it. If you're unclear, admit it. She doesn't need perfection; she needs presence. She needs to know you won't disappear the moment your ego is hurt.

Honesty doesn't make you weak. It makes you trustworthy. A man who can speak the truth when it costs him is a man who can be counted on when it matters most.

July 24th

Make Her Feel Chosen Daily

A masculine man doesn't just say she's the one; you show it. You show it in how you listen without distractions, in how your eyes lock on hers when she speaks, and in how your presence silences her doubt before it ever needs words.

You pay attention to her rhythms, her stress, and her softness, and you meet her without needing her to ask. You walk past her in the kitchen and touch her lower back. You pull her in and kiss her after a long day. You send the message without ever saying it:

You're mine. I see you. I choose you. Still. Always.

Action:

1. Daily Contact: Create a moment each day where she feels held, even if it's just a 15-second kiss with nothing else behind it.

2. Unprompted Gesture: Do one small thing for her without her asking. Bring her a drink. Run her bath. Touch her hair while she reads.

3. Eye Contact: Stop. Look at her. Hold it for three full breaths. Say nothing. Just let her feel chosen in your gaze.

July 25th

Gain Influence in Every Room

When the foundation of your relationship is grounded in love, not chaos or control, it radiates something most can't fake: stability.

The way you walk, the calmness in your presence, the respect she reflects - it all speaks before you do. People watch. They sense your alignment and your integrity, and whether it's in business or social settings, your energy becomes influential.

When you lead a woman well, you signal that you can lead yourself. When you can lead yourself, people will follow, not out of fear but out of deep, unspoken respect.

In a world of performance, grounded masculine love is rare. Rare earns influence without needing to demand it.

July 26th

Learn to Lead in the Bedroom

Masculine presence doesn't wait for permission; it reads the moment and acts with certainty. Leading in the bedroom isn't about dominance for ego. It's about direction rooted in a deep connection.

She doesn't want to map it out or coach you through it. She wants to feel your awareness. Your patience. Your intensity. She wants to relax into her feminine, but only when she knows you've got the wheel.

Action:

1. Tonight, lead without words.
2. Create the atmosphere, low lights, slow music, and intention in your touch.
3. Watch her breath, her micro-movements, her reactions.
4. Adjust in real time. Don't rush. Don't perform.

July 27th

You Experience Peace at Home

A masculine man doesn't bring the chaos of the world into his home; he leaves it at the door. He understands that his presence sets the emotional climate. When he walks in, his energy either tightens the room or softens it.

You don't wait for calm to happen; you cultivate it through consistency. Through presence. Through clear communication and emotional responsibility. You don't raise your voice to be heard. You ground your tone to be understood. You listen, not to react, but to connect. That alone defuses tension.

Your woman leans into you not just for pleasure but for restoration. The kids look to you not with far but with admiration, and when you're alone, there's no internal conflict because your life is aligned. The house becomes more than a shelter; it becomes a sanctuary. Not because everything is perfect but because you show up with strength wrapped in steadiness.

July 28th

Get the Right Woman, Not Just Any Woman

A masculine man doesn't scatter his energy to feel validated. You refine your standard, live your values, and let your presence do the filtering. When your life is anchored in purpose, discipline, and direction, you stop needing to impress and start magnetising the woman who truly sees you.

She doesn't just want the image; she wants the reality. She wants a man with depth, a mission, an edge, and a purpose.

Action:

1. Audit who you give your time, attention, and desire to.
2. Stop entertaining women who drain, distract, or derail your path, especially if they're beautiful. That false dopamine costs your long-term clarity.
3. Replace chasing with building. Get sharp on what you're creating. Build a life where a high-calibre woman doesn't need saving or being impressed but is honoured and respected for who she is.
4. Be the man she's proud to stand beside, not because you chased her, but because you stood tall enough to meet her at her level.

July 29th

Your Children Learn from Your Example

Your son watches how you show up daily, how you move through pressure, and how you lead with both power and presence. That's how he defines manhood, not by what you say but by what you embody.

Your daughter watches even closer. She reads your tone, your eyes, and your energy. That's what sets her standard, not for fantasy but for safety, leadership, and devotion.

What you model becomes their inner compass. Don't aim to raise strong kids, be the strong man they mirror. Make love visible. Make boundaries felt. Let them witness absolute integrity, real patience, and real power in motion.

July 30th

Grow Together or Grow Apart

Love isn't something you win once and then leave on autopilot. It requires presence, pulse checks, and playful tension. If you're not growing together, you're growing apart.

Check-in not just when there's a problem but also when things are going well. Are you both stretching yourselves too thin? Do your values still align? Are you both still seen and lit up by one another?

Here's where your masculine leadership deepens; you keep the edge alive. You take the date night off autopilot. You plan spontaneous adventures. You flirt, tease, and claim her like it's day one, with the depth of year ten.

Keep the mystery alive, not by withholding love, but by continually evolving. Keep fun alive, not with gimmicks, but with presence. Keep sex alive, not through pressure, but through playful polarity.

Relationships fail when men fall asleep at the wheel. Masculine love says: "I'll keep showing up, growing, checking in, reigniting the fire, because I don't just want you in my life. I want us to keep rising together."

July 31st

Don't Just Love, You Transform

Masculine love isn't passive. It's not about comfort, convenience, or coasting. It's about creation. You don't just show up for her; you rise for her. You don't just give her affection; you ignite her evolution. She doesn't settle into you; she expands because of you.

True masculine love is an amplifier. It turns moments into memories, chemistry into depth, sex into sacred fire. It doesn't dim either of you; it refines both of you. Your love becomes the container where her feminine energy flourishes, her guard drops, and her full expression unlocks.

In that same space, you sharpen, too. You lead clearly. Listen deeper. Trust stronger. You elevate not just as a man but as a partner, father, and legacy builder. When masculine love is real, it doesn't just feel good; it is good. It's intentional and about holding space with strength, leading with integrity, and loving so deeply that it reshapes both of your lives.

You don't chase love. You become the kind of man that love can't help but stay with.

August

Connection & Flow

Find Your State. Move with Nature, People, and Power

Learn to connect to something far more profound than just goals or noise. It's about dropping into your true masculine state, where your body, mind, and environment operate as one.

The modern masculine man doesn't isolate. You integrate. You read energy, lead from alignment, and move with rhythm, not resistance. Flow isn't passive; it's powerful. It's the sharp calm behind the action. The stillness before the strike. The awareness that turns instinct into impact.

You'll learn to connect to nature, not for escape, but for recalibration. You'll learn to connect to others, not to be liked, but to lead, and you'll learn to connect to yourself, so you stop reacting to life and start guiding it.

This month, you'll find that your most significant edge doesn't come from force; it comes from flow, and the man who can drop into his zone on command becomes dangerous. Because while others are chasing control, you're riding the wave your way.

"True power isn't in force; it's in alignment. A masculine man moves with life, not against it."

August 1st

Presence Is Power

Your ability to be fully present, without distraction or agenda, is the foundation of deep connection. It's not about what you say. It's not about what you do. It's how you are in the room.

A woman knows when you're fully with her. She feels it in your eye contact, in your breathing, in the way your energy doesn't drift. In business, people follow the man who is grounded in the present, not scattered across thoughts, worries, or checking a screen every ten seconds. Presence commands without raising your voice.

In a world that's addicted to noise, the man who chooses stillness becomes rare and respected.

Action: (5 Minutes Daily)

1. Choose the moment: Before a conversation, a date, or even a meeting, take 5 minutes to ground yourself. No phone. No agenda.
2. Sit still and observe your breath: Inhale slowly through your nose, exhale slowly through your mouth. Drop your shoulders.

3. Focus your attention: Select one sound in the environment or a sensation in your body. Stay with it. When the mind wanders, gently bring it back to focus.

4. Walk into the interaction with one intention: Be here fully. Not half. Not distracted. Fully.

5. Practice presence under pressure: The next time you're speaking to someone and feel the urge to interrupt, solve, or prove, pause. Breathe. Listen. Stay.

August 2nd

Enhanced Relationships

A deep connection isn't about harm or convenience; it's rooted in truth, presence, and mutual respect. A masculine man who lives in flow doesn't force connection; you cultivate it. You listen without needing to fix everything. You speak without ego. You hold space without control.

Women feel safer. Friends feel seen. Business allies feel understood because you're not just showing up physically; you're with them energetically. When your presence is real, and your word is grounded, relationships don't drain you; they fuel you. They become an extension of your clarity and strength. You attract people who are aligned, not just available, and that's where trust, intimacy, and loyalty multiply.

August 3rd

Stillness Is Strength

In a chaotic world, everyone is reacting, chasing, and proving. The masculine man who cultivates stillness becomes magnetic. Not passive, powerful. His energy doesn't scatter. It anchors.

Stillness isn't silence. Its presence with weight. It's the clarity in your eyes when others flinch. The control of your breath when others spiral. The grounded edge that makes people lean in, not because you're loud, but because you don't need to be.

Women feel safe in that space. Men respect it, and life responds to it because true strength is in how unshakable you remain when the storm hits.

August 4th

Emotional Resilience

True masculine power isn't about suppressing emotions; it's about holding them with discipline. The emotionally resilient man doesn't explode, collapse, or run. You absorb. You process, and you act with precision.

Life will throw chaos at you in business, relationships, and your mind. The man with emotional resilience doesn't lose his edge. You breathe through conflict. You listen when triggered. You lead through pressure. That composure becomes your weapon and your anchor.

Emotional resilience isn't natural; it's trained, and once mastered, it becomes the difference between a man who survives and one who leads through the storm.

Action:

1. Name the emotion: Don't just feel "off." Identify the following emotions: anger, shame, overwhelm, and fear. Naming gives clarity.
2. Breathe deeply through the nose for 2 minutes: This reactivates presence and dampens emotional reactivity.
3. Ask one high-level question: "What's the opportunity in this?" or "What's the lesson I need right now?"

4. Move your body: Do push-ups, go for a sprint, or take a cold shower. Don't sit in emotion. Transmute it through motion.

5. Choose an aligned action: Decide with clarity, not chaos. Respond from leadership, not reaction.

August 5th

Nature Is Your Mirror

The masculine man doesn't conquer nature; you listen to it. The way you respond to nature is the way you react to life. Fast or still. Forceful or flowing. Focused or scattered.

The ocean doesn't rush. The mountain doesn't apologise. The tree doesn't chase.

When you align with nature's pace, you start to recognise your rhythms, your triggers, your tensions, and your truths. You see clearly what's real and what's noise.

Nature reveals that if you're anxious, you'll resist its stillness. If you're grounded, you'll move with its flow, not softly but by being aware. A high-level man who understands an emotional landscape doesn't just feel; he deciphers. You see the link between your inner world and your actions. Between your breath and your power.

When your energy is chaotic, go outside and take a walk. Touch the earth. Sit with the wind. Let your body sync to Mother Earth's tempo, not your phone's. Masculine presence sharpens in nature.

August 6th

Increased Self-Awareness

Understanding your inner world is not optional for the masculine man; it's foundational. Masculine strength lives in clarity, and clarity only comes when you learn to observe yourself, not through judgment but through precision.

You start to notice:

When your energy drops after a particular conversation.

When your patience slips under specific pressure.

When you shift from a grounded to a reactive state.

When you reach for distraction instead of discipline.

Being self-aware becomes your edge, not just for peace but for power, because the man who knows his patterns can shape them. The man who recognises his triggers can reroute them. The man who understands his emotional blueprint can build relationships, business, and legacy without sabotaging himself from the inside.

Increased self-awareness means you stop living on default. You stop leaking energy, and you stop lying to yourself. You start making decisions that are yours, rooted in purpose rather than old programming. Once you master that, everything else falls into place.

August 7th

Balance Doing with Being

The high-level masculine man knows when to push and when to pause, but most men burn out trying to do more. They confuse movement with progress. Doing without presence becomes chaos masked as productivity. That's not power, that's depletion.

True masculine flow is a rhythm. Drive paired with depth. Movement anchored in meaning. You're not here to hustle endlessly. You're here to move with precision. To act from alignment, not urgency.

Balancing doing with being doesn't make you softer; it makes you strategic. It lends weight to your words, presence to your actions, and peace to your pursuit. The man who knows how to stop is the man who never truly loses his edge.

Action:

1. Morning Clarity (10 min): Before doing anything, sit still. No phone. No input. Just you, your breath, and one question: "What matters today?"
2. Midday Reset (5–10 min): Halfway through your day, take a silent walk. No headphones. No agenda. Reconnect with nature or your breath. Let your nervous system reset.

3. Evening Reflection (10 min): Reflect on your day with honesty. Did I lead with presence or chase tasks? Did I connect or perform? Adjust accordingly.

August 8th

Cultivate Deep Listening

Masculine strength is shown in action and felt in stillness. One of the rarest masculine traits today is the ability to listen truly. Not just to respond. Not just to fix. But to understand.

When a man listens with their full presence, without judgment, without interruption, and ego, others open up. Women soften. Men respect your leadership, and it becomes magnetic, without force, because deep listening shows one thing louder than words ever could: I see you. I'm here.

In a world addicted to speaking, the man who listens wins. When your woman or your tribe knows you hear them, they follow you with loyalty, not resistance.

Action:

1. When someone speaks, pause briefly before replying. Let the words land.
2. Mirror back a key phrase: "What I hear you saying is…"
3. Drop the urge to solve; first, sit with it. That alone often dissolves more tension than solutions do.
4. This is followed by processing the conversation and its outcome to identify how it differed.

August 9th

Greater Life Satisfaction

Satisfaction is achieved when your actions align with your values, when your daily rhythm resonates with your purpose, and when your private and public selves are in harmony.

You wake up knowing what you're building. You look in the mirror and respect the man looking back. You move through the world, not needing to prove but ready to serve.

That's the real edge: when your ambition has meaning—allowing fulfilment that doesn't fade with applause or collapse when things go quiet. You're not just living; you're living in alignment. That's where masculine satisfaction isn't just felt; it's embodied.

August 10th

Balanced Energy

True masculine power isn't about endless output; it's about intelligent rhythm, and when you learn to harmonise action with rest, pressure with pause, and intensity with recovery, you stop burning out and start building long-term fire.

You move like a man who chooses his pace, not by fear or the need to prove. You train hard, and then you recover. You lead boldly, and then you unplug. You give deeply from a full cup.

This balance isn't about softness; it's about strategy. When your nervous system is steady, your decisions are cleaner. Your body performs better. Your relationships deepen. Your leadership sharpens.

Masculine energy that's always "on" becomes scattered and drained.

Calibrated masculine energy becomes focused and magnetic. That's the edge, not just having energy but mastering its flow.

August 11th

Authentic Leadership

The masculine man leads from a grounded centre, not a bloated ego. You don't need titles or applause. Your influence comes from empathy, integrity, and presence. People feel safe around you, not because you control but because you understand.

Authentic leadership is about congruence. Who you are in private matches who you are in public. Your team, your woman, your children, they know what to expect. That's rare. That's powerful.

You don't bark. You build.

You don't manipulate. You model.

You don't push from fear. You pull from purpose.

In a world of performers, the man who leads with integrity becomes the one others trust to follow.

Action:

1. Pick one area, your business, your relationship, or your friend group and lead it from empathy instead of ego.
2. Ask questions before issuing orders.
3. Listen longer than usual.

4. Be decisive but also aware of how your choices are perceived.
5. Watch how respect grows when presence leads the way.

August 12th

Honour Your Intuition

The masculine man doesn't just think clearly; he senses deeply. Intuition is precision. It's your internal compass that operates beneath logic. While strategy maps the terrain, intuition tells you when to move.

The world teaches men to overvalue logic and suppress feelings. True strength lies in integrating both. Intuition sharpens timing, reveals hidden truths, and keeps you aligned when facts alone aren't enough. It's how you know who to trust, when to pivot, and where the energy is shifting.

You've felt it before: That quiet nudge to walk away from a deal that looked perfect. The knowing that your woman wasn't okay, even when she said she was.

That's not a coincidence. That's your more profound wisdom, and when you honour intuition, your leadership deepens. Your relationships sharpen. Your flow strengthens. You're no longer just operating; you're aligned.

August 13th

Foster Authentic Relationships

Genuine masculine connection holds truth, not performance. You don't build lasting bonds by impressing; you make them by being real. Authentic relationships grow when you drop the armour and show up with presence, honesty, and respect. Masculine men don't fear vulnerability; they lead with it wisely.

Surface-level talk creates surface-level trust, and when you speak from depth, when you're willing to own your truth and invite the same from others, something shifts. That's when loyalty forms. That's when love deepens. That's when brotherhood solidifies.

A masculine connection doesn't need to be loud or constant; it just needs to be genuine. From that place, your relationships stop draining you and start refuelling you.

Action:

1. Initiate one real conversation this week: Ask a close friend or partner, "What's something you're carrying right now that no one sees?" Then, listen fully without solving or judging.

2. Share something you've been withholding: Not for attention, but for clarity. Lead with, "Here's something

I haven't said, but I feel it's time." Watch how the bond sharpens.

3. Audit your circle: Who do you feel comfortable being real with? Who are you still performing for? Begin shifting your energy away from facades and toward truth.

August 14th

Enhanced Creativity

For the masculine man, creativity isn't just about producing ideas; it's about perceiving more profound truths. Flow state removes noise and activates pattern recognition: the ability to see what others miss, connect dots others overlook, and act on insights before the rest even notice the signals.

This level of creativity isn't chaotic; it's refined. In flow, your nervous system is calm, your mind is sharp, and your awareness expands. You're not reacting. You're reading. Sensing. Integrating. You start noticing recurring themes in conversations, market shifts in business, and emotional cycles in relationships, and you move with precision.

You become the man who builds what others thought was impossible—the man who says the thing that hits the nerve. You solve the problem before it becomes a crisis.

Creativity guided by pattern recognition isn't guesswork; it's mastery. It's a masculine power that merges instinct with execution. When you're connected to that source, you don't just express ideas; you shape reality.

August 15th

Practice Mindful Communication

For the masculine man, words are not weapons or fillers; they are instruments of influence. Mindful communication means you speak from awareness, not reaction. You choose your tone, your timing, and your truth with precision.

You don't dump your emotions.

You don't dominate the space.

You create a channel where clarity leads, and confusion ends.

Shifting relational dynamics. In partnership, your woman leans in because she feels seen and safe, not spoken over or dismissed. In business, you become the man whose words carry weight, not noise. With friends, you build trust because you listen to understand, not just to respond.

When you practice mindful communication:

1. You slow your breath before you speak
2. You feel the energy in the room
3. You ask yourself: "What creates a connection here?"
4. You don't rush to fill the silence; you let it sharpen your presence

August 16th

Integrate Masculine and Feminine Energies

A high-level masculine man isn't just force; he's fusion. You lead with direction but listen with presence. You take action and know when to surrender. You hold boundaries but also have space. That's what makes you rare. That's what makes you trusted.

The modern world teaches men to overemphasise logic, aggression, and control without intuition, stillness, and awareness. Without these qualities, you become rigid, reactive, and eventually burned out. The real edge is in balance.

The most dangerous man in the room is the one who can build and receive, assert, and feel, penetrate, and protect, all in one breath.

Action: (15 minutes)

1. Track your last week: Write down five moments where you responded to a challenge or conversation.

   Were you reactive or receptive? Did you push, or did you pause and sense?

2. Identify your imbalance: Are you overly assertive but emotionally disconnected?

Or overly empathetic but passive in direction? Call it out clearly.

3. Daily integration practice

In one situation today, lead with clarity (masculine)

In another, receive fully without speaking (feminine)

Reflect nightly on what felt powerful and what felt unfamiliar

August 17th

Prioritise Self-Care

Too many men wear burnout like a badge, grinding until the tank is empty, relationships strain, and clarity fades. That's not power. That's slow self-destruction. High-level masculine energy isn't about running until you collapse; it's about maintaining your edge so you can give more without breaking and more efficiently.

Self-care isn't a weakness. It's a strategy. When you are well-rested, deeply nourished, and mentally clear, your presence becomes magnetic. You respond instead of reacting. You feel, instead of being numb. You lead with more charge, more trust, and more depth.

The masculine man doesn't wait until he breaks to care for himself. You stay ahead of the fall. When you operate from a foundation of strength and stability, the connection isn't forced; it flows.

Action:

1. Set a non-negotiable workout schedule: Train not to escape but to sharpen.
2. Protect your sleep as if your success depends on it because it does.

3. Unplug one hour daily, no devices, breathe, space, stillness, or reflection.

4. Fuel like a warrior, eat clean, hydrate deeply, and move like you mean it.

5. Honour your mental health by journaling, meditating, or seeking guidance before the crisis hits.

August 18th

Engage in Continuous Learning

In a world that's evolving by the second, stagnation is a death sentence. True masculine power isn't locked in a moment; it adapts, refines, and expands. You don't need to know everything, but you must be relentless in your pursuit of learning. From books, mentors, failures, feedback, the feminine, and the stillness of nature, growth is everywhere for the man who is awake to it.

When you commit to continuous learning, you sharpen your mind, deepen your emotional intelligence, and broaden your spiritual bandwidth. You become a man who responds, not reacts. Who evolves, not erodes?

Masculine men don't just seek mastery in skill; they seek mastery in self. That growth doesn't just make you adaptable. It makes you magnetic. It deepens your connection to others because your presence carries wisdom, not just knowledge.

The man who is always learning becomes the man who is always leading.

Action:

1. Choose one domain to sharpen each week: mental, physical, emotional, relational, or spiritual.

2. Read or listen 30 minutes a day from high-level thinkers, leaders, or teachers outside your comfort zone.

3. Ask for feedback from someone you trust, especially when you resist hearing it.

4. Track what challenged you most each week, then learn from it, not judge it.

August 19th

Stronger Intuition

Intuition is the silent intelligence behind decisive action. It's not emotional guessing; it's the refined perception that comes from being fully connected to yourself, your environment, and your experiences. It's the voice beneath the noise that tells you this is right, or this is off, long before logic catches up.

For the high-level masculine man, strong intuition shines through presence, awareness, and repetition. You train it the way you train your body by listening, testing, and refining, and when it's sharp, it becomes your edge in relationships, business, leadership, and life.

You'll know who to trust before they prove it.

You'll feel when your woman's energy shifts without her saying a word.

You'll make the right decision before the facts present themselves.

You'll move before others even notice the opportunity.

Men lead without force; they're in rhythm with reality. Strengthen your intuition by staying grounded, reducing mental clutter, and honouring the messages your body and instincts send. The more you trust yourself, the more life starts aligning in your favour.

The man who trusts his inner voice walks with clarity, and everyone around him can feel it.

August 20th

Personal Growth

Growth doesn't happen by accident. It's intentional. A masculine man understands you're not just building muscle or status; you're refining your inner framework. Personal growth is the relentless pursuit of becoming sharper, wiser, and more grounded. It's knowing that who you are today is not the final version; it's the current baseline.

This kind of growth requires humility and a relentless pursuit of more. You stop reacting to life and start responding with intelligence and purpose. You seek out feedback. You question old beliefs. You track your patterns. You do the inner work not for applause but for alignment.

As you grow, everything else grows with you.

Your relationship deepens.

Your business becomes smoother.

Your presence becomes magnetic.

You start leading from essence, not ego.

The masculine man doesn't fear growth; you pursue it like a code of honour. Staying the same is a silent form of betrayal to the man you're capable of becoming.

Action: (15 Minutes Every Sunday Night)

1. Review Your Week: What worked? What didn't? Don't judge, observe.

2. Track Patterns: Where did the same frustration or reaction show up again?

3. Set One Growth Intention: Choose one area, mindset, habit, or relationship to level up this week.

4. Integrate One Tool: Read, apply, or test one new idea, technique, or perspective.

5. Lock It In: Write down a one-line statement that defines how you'll move this week differently.

August 21st

Set Healthy Boundaries

Boundaries aren't walls. They're standards. They define where your energy ends and where someone else's begins. When you set healthy boundaries, you're not being selfish; you're being sovereign. You're choosing what enters your space, your mind, and your time.

You're not pushing people away. It's about letting the right ones come closer in the right way. The masculine man doesn't allow his peace to be taken by guilt, obligation, or manipulation. He knows that access to him is earned, not assumed.

People respect you more. Women trust you deeply. Friends lean on you but don't lean too hard. Healthy boundaries elevate your leadership. You stop leaking energy into people-pleasing and start channelling it into purpose. Your presence becomes cleaner. Your life becomes simpler. Your relationships become clearer.

Setting boundaries isn't a rejection of others. It's a declaration of self-respect. It's how you protect your mission, honour your values, and stay grounded while the world pulls you in every direction.

August 22nd

Spiritual Fulfillment

Spiritual fulfilment isn't about religion; it's about alignment. A deep, internal connection to meaning. A knowing that your life has weight, not just in what you do, but in how you show up.

When a man connects to the larger rhythm, to nature, to the universe, to creation itself, you stop chasing significance and start living it—your ego quiets. Your actions carry reverence. You see your path not as random but as intentional. Guided.

Empowering you to stop forcing outcomes. You're reading the signals. You're moving in harmony with a higher current. People feel that presence. It's calming. It's clarifying. It's commanding.

Spiritual fulfilment isn't a destination; it's a daily alignment. The masculine man who walks in this clarity moves with unmatched conviction. You don't need applause. You've already heard the call.

When you lead from this place, life opens in ways force never could.

Action: (Daily – 10 Minutes)

1. Start with Stillness: Sit or stand outdoors, if possible. Breathe deeply. Feel your body. No distractions.

2. Ask One Question: "What am I here to give today?" Sit with it. Don't force an answer. Let it arise.

3. Feel Connection: Visualise your place in the bigger picture. The people you impact. The legacy you're shaping.

4. Anchor It in Action: Decide one thing you'll do today to serve that higher purpose, even if it's small. Do it deliberately.

August 23rd

Lead with Integrity

When a man leads with integrity, you become unshakable. Your words match your actions. Your decisions align with your values, and people follow because they trust you.

Integrity means doing the right thing when it's hard when no one's watching, and when it costs you. It's not about being perfect. It's about being principled, and in a world flooded with noise and performance, that kind of clarity cuts through everything.

Women feel safe under your leadership. Men, take your word seriously. Teams, families, and movements gather around you because they know this man holds the line. You don't fall apart under pressure. You don't chase applause. You build a legacy, one aligned step at a time.

August 24th

Embody Gratitude

To embody gratitude is to move through life fully present, grounded in appreciation for both the wins and the wounds. The masculine man doesn't just list what he's thankful for; he lives it. Your energy radiates presence because you're not waiting for the future to validate you. You're already rich in awareness.

Gratitude brings calm to chaos, clarity to confusion, and connection to isolation. It reframes setbacks as training grounds. It turns discomfort into refinement. It roots you so deeply in the now that external noise can't shake you.

When you embody gratitude, people feel safer around you. Women lean in. Men respect you, and life begins to open up to you with more opportunities. Not because you asked but because you've become the kind of man who notices.

Action:

1. Start each day by physically grounding yourself, barefoot on earth, one hand on heart, one on breath.

2. Speak three things out loud that you are genuinely grateful for, not surface-level, but real.

3. Carry that awareness into your interactions. Slow your pace. Look people in the eye.

4. Acknowledge the small moments, the warmth of sunlight, the strength in your body, and the lesson from yesterday's mistake.

August 25th

Improved Physical Health

A masculine man aligned in thought, breath, and movement doesn't just look healthy; he is. It's about cultivating a body that performs, recovers, and endures with precision. When you operate from a state of presence, gratitude, and internal clarity, your nervous system relaxes. Stress drops. Hormones regulate. Sleep deepens. Inflammation lowers. Recovery accelerates.

Your training becomes smarter. Your nutrition becomes more intuitive, and your physical energy becomes consistent, not fluctuating, but strong, focused, and grounded. Mind-body alignment is surgical. It allows you to push harder without breaking because you're not battling your system. You're aligning it.

Your requirement to dominate long-term in your career, relationship, and legacy.

August 26th

Emotional Balance

A masculine man doesn't explode. He doesn't collapse. He stays grounded in pressure, calm in chaos, and centred in uncertainty. Emotional balance means you feel deeply without being ruled by the feeling. You hold space for anger without reacting to it. You process pain without projecting it. You can be passionate without being unstable.

That's the difference between power and volatility. Between being a presence to be relied on or a fuse walked on.

Inner harmony is the understanding of your emotional triggers, recognising patterns, and choosing a response over a reaction. That choice, repeated daily, sharpens your clarity, deepens your relationships, and earns trust, especially with women, because she feels safe. Not because you're emotionless but because you don't lose yourself in emotion. You become a man whose internal world is steady, and that steadiness becomes your advantage everywhere.

August 27th

Your Integrity Becomes
Your Identity

A masculine man doesn't live for applause. He lives aligned. Your actions echo long after your voice is gone. Integrity means your name carries weight in rooms you've never walked into. It's how your woman speaks about you when you're not there. It's what your children model without needing to be told. It's the quiet standard you set that others elevate to meet.

You don't just inspire by what you do but by who you consistently are. In your business, your relationships, your fatherhood, and your private thoughts. Integrity builds trust, and trust builds a legacy. Not a legacy of noise but of depth. The kind of legacy that roots itself in people's lives and lifts them.

Your wealth can fade. Your strength can fade. Your integrity remains solid in the hearts of those who felt your presence and saw your consistency.

August 28th

Align Your Rhythm with the Environment

Nature holds a rhythm older than time, and when you ignore it, you fall into friction. Burnout. Confusion. Delay. When you rise with the sun, train with the tide, and move with intention through the day, you begin to operate like a force of nature, grounded, precise, and instinctively effective.

You eat when your body calls, not when a clock tells you. You sleep when recovery is needed, not when the hustle culture says you're weak. You work in alignment with your natural peak states, your creativity, your physical power, and your emotional clarity. You stop managing time like a machine and start honouring energy like a warrior.

Masculine flow isn't laziness. It's an efficient action. It's knowing that timing matters more than effort. It's understanding you don't need to kick open every door, and timing plays its part. That's leadership. That's presence.

When you live in this present, aligned, and responsive state, life moves smoothly. You don't chase. You attract. You're no longer the man trying to keep up. You're the one others are trying to read.

August 29th

Become a Channel, Not a Container

Masculine flow isn't about holding it all in; it's about letting it move through you. Energy, wisdom, emotion, presence, these aren't trophies to collect. They're currents to the channel. The immature man holds. The masculine man transmits. When you become a channel, life stops feeling heavy. You stop clutching for control and start moving with precision, power, and peace.

Containers overflow. Channelers circulate. That's the difference between burnout and embodiment.

You're not here to store knowledge, to hoard power, to flex your emotional control like a fortress. You're here to be a vessel of alignment, strong enough to hold your own, open enough to share it. When you live this way, you don't just make an impact; you ignite it.

Action:

1. Emotionally: Speak something real today. One truth you've been sitting on. Say it clean. Say it calmly. Don't let it rot inside you.

2. Physically: Move energy through your body. Breathwork, sprinting, lifting, and cold plunge. Get it moving; don't let it stagnate.

3. Spiritually: Share insight. Teach one thing you've learned. Don't wait to be perfect. Circulate what's alive in you now.

4. Energetically: Touch someone's life today without needing recognition. Your presence is powerful; use it.

Find Silence Between the Signals

In a world that overvalues noise, productivity, and constant output, it's the man who can sit in silence and become dangerous because he hears what others miss. Between every success and setback is a signal. Between every emotional pull is an instruction. Between every inhale and exhale lies a moment of total presence if you're brave enough to feel its depth, direction, and clarity in the natural rhythm of the masculine flow.

The man who leads with grace doesn't guess. You tune in with grounded certainty. You recognise that clarity doesn't scream; it whispers. To hear it, you must be still enough to listen. You become the one others follow, not because you're loud but because you move with the truth.

August 31st

Connection Begins with Self-Containment

Before you connect deeply with others, with purpose, or with the world, you must connect fully with yourself. Masculine power doesn't leak. It contains. It holds its line, its energy, its presence. That containment isn't a restriction; it's clarity. It's knowing where you begin and end. It's knowing what emotions are yours and what's just noise. It's honouring your edges, your values, and your rhythms without guilt, apology, or collapse.

When your inner world is clear, your outer world responds. Conversations sharpen. Leadership becomes effortless. You stop seeking validation and start emanating a grounded presence, one that commands a state of flow.

Flow doesn't emerge from scattered energy; it requires alignment. It requires a body that's regulated. A mind that's focused, and emotions that are integrated, not repressed. When you are self-contained, the flow becomes your default.

Benefits of Flow State for the Masculine Man:

1. Sharper decisions under pressure: Distractions are gone
2. More impact with fewer words: Your energy speaks first

3. Heightened attraction: Your presence is magnetic

4. Stronger leadership: You respond, not react

5. Deepened intimacy: She can finally feel you, not your chaos

6. Sustained performance: You're not burning out; you're tuned in

September

Power & Enterprise

Build. Dominate. Lead. The Masculine Code of Business

Step onto the battlefield of modern enterprise with the mindset of a warrior, calculated, dangerous, and decisive. Business isn't just about strategy; it's psychological warfare, and your edge is how you present yourself: clear, controlled, and with complete confidence.

Don't chase money; build powerful structures. Systems that reflect your discipline. Income that demonstrates your impact. Leadership that leaves no doubt. The masculine man doesn't just hustle; he executes with intent, leads with presence, and negotiates from a position of purpose.

You'll learn how to move like a boardroom savage: when to speak, when to watch, when to strike. You'll learn how to build deals with precision, stand in rooms where pressure is currency, and expand without apology. You don't just make a business; you're building your name. You don't follow trends; you're building a legacy.

This month is about stepping into your complete masculine enterprise, where your ambition is weaponised, your decisions are clear, and your path is designed, not dictated.

"A man doesn't chase opportunity; he builds it, owns it, and walks in with leverage."

Own the Room Before You Speak

The man who owns the room doesn't need to announce himself; your presence speaks before your mouth opens. Your posture is upright, your eyes are steady, your energy is grounded, and you are not looking for attention; you already have it.

There is no arrogance; it's authority grounded in self-trust. You walk in clear on who you are, what you stand for, and what you bring. No need to over-express, outshine, or prove. That certainty is rare, which is why it's notable.

People respect the man who can hold silence without tension, who listens fully before speaking, who speaks with precision, not noise. In every boardroom, gym, stage, or conversation, the man who owns the room is the one who's already owned himself.

You don't own the room because you're the loudest. You own it because your energy is undeniable.

Action:

1. Walk In With Breath, Not Bravado: Before entering any room, take three deep nasal breaths to ground your energy. Show up calm, not hyped.

2. Posture Check: The spine is tall, the shoulders are back, and the chin is level. You are commanding space, not collapsing into it.

3. Make Eye Contact With Intention: Look at people directly and maintain the gaze without force. One second longer than comfortable. That's where respect is born.

4. Speak Less, Say More: Cut filler words. When you speak, slow down. Every word lands with more weight.

5. Stay Unshaken: If challenged, don't react; take a deep breath and remain calm. A masculine man doesn't defend his worth. He stands in it.

Stop Pitching, Start Positioning

Masculine business isn't about begging for attention. It's about becoming the man whose presence creates demand. When you pitch, you're chasing. When you position, you pull. High-level operators, partners, and clients don't respond to desperation; they respond to direction.

Positioning is a silent strength. It's how you show up. It's the energy in your presence, the clarity in your message, the alignment between what you say and how you live. Masculine men don't overexplain; they embody. You don't need to convince people when your life reflects your values.

Action:

1. Audit Your Online Presence: Google your name. Look at your socials. Would you invest in yourself? Would your presence command respect without a pitch? Identify what needs upgrading.

2. Clarify Your One-Liner: Define exactly who you are, what you solve, and who it's for — in one clear, confident sentence. No fluff. All weight.

3. Stand for One Thing: Stop being broad. Be known for one dominant value or outcome. Precision cuts through the noise.

4. Refine Your Image: Dress like the leader you are. Speak like every word matters. Move with certainty. People buy the man before they buy the offer.

5. Own Your Space: Show up in the right rooms, then speak less. Hold posture, eye contact, and grounded energy. You're not there to take; you're there to be chosen.

September 3rd

Move in Silence Until You Strike

Masculine strategy is subtle. You don't need to broadcast your every move; you need to build it with intention. The man of power isn't loud about his plans. You refine them. Strengthen them, and sharpen yourself in the dark, so when you move, it's precise and unstoppable.

Silence isn't a weakness; it's a form of calibration. It keeps distractions out and energy focused. While others overshare, overexpose, and seek validation, you're building assets, refining your vision, and becoming undeniable —not through noise, but through results.

When you strike, in business, in life, in any arena, it's clean. Effective. Respected. It wasn't a reactive move; it was a calculated and quiet execution. Be the storm they never saw coming.

Action:

1. Guard Your Intentions: Don't reveal your next move— power leaks through over-sharing.
2. Refine Your Craft Daily: Build what matters behind closed doors. Use solitude to sharpen skills and amplify clarity.

3. Limit Outside Voices: Everyone has an opinion. Fewer should have access. Silence helps filter noise from the truth.

4. Let Results Speak: Make excellence your announcement. When you land the deal, release the product, or shift the room, that's your proof.

5. Strike With Precision: When you move, do so with complete intention. No half-effort. No hesitation. Your strike should feel inevitable.

September 4th

Be a Value Creator, Not a Time Drainer

Masculine presence doesn't consume; it contributes. You walk into a room, and people feel elevated. Not because you demand attention but because your energy, words, and actions offer something rare: value.

Weak men take time, ask for energy, and drain the space. Masculine men give. They solve problems, refine ideas, and advance the mission. Whether it's a relationship, a business table, or a brotherhood, your presence either builds momentum or breaks it.

A high-value man doesn't need to beg for seats at the table. He becomes indispensable at it. Your time is a currency, but your value is the brand you represent. Don't chase validation. Deliver so much value that they chase you.

Action:

1. Audit Your Interactions: After every meeting or conversation, ask yourself, "Did I bring clarity, energy, or strategy?" If not, adjust.

2. Study the Room: Listen more than you speak. Find the gap and fill it.

3. Upgrade Your Language: Speak in solutions, not stories. Eliminate the filler. Make every word serve a purpose.

4. Add Energy, Don't Steal It: When you show up, bring grounded momentum. Avoid projecting neediness, complaints, or drama.

5. Build Your Toolbox: Acquire New Skills. Refine your offers. The more you can do, the more you can give. That's masculine leverage.

September 5th

Your Network is a Mirror, Upgrade It

Masculine evolution isn't just about what you build; it's about who you make it with. The men you surround yourself with reflect your standards, your vision, and your future. If they're soft, unfocused, or constantly circling comfort, that energy seeps into you.

A powerful man curates his circle as if his empire depends on it because it does. Strong networks level you up. They challenge your excuses. They pose better questions, and they move in alignment, not driven by emotion. In high-level masculine spaces, iron sharpens iron, or it gets removed.

Every conversation either sharpens your direction or dulls your drive. Your circle is either a ceiling or a launchpad. Choose accordingly. As a masculine man, your future has seats. The question is: who's sitting with you?

Action:

1. Audit Your Top 5: Write down the five people you spend the most time with. Are they building? Are they growing? Do they call you out or keep you safe?

2. Drop the Drainers: Identify who always complains, gossips, or keeps you small. You don't need drama dressed as friendship. Quietly limit access.

3. Seek Strategic Proximity: Join rooms that challenge your thinking. Find mentors, masterminds, or tribes that challenge your baseline.

4. Lead with Value: Don't network to take advantage of others. Network to contribute. Show up with clarity, energy, and usefulness, and watch doors open.

5. Upgrade Your Conversations: Focus on talking less about others. More talk about mission, money, energy, legacy, and impact. That's how high-level men connect.

Money is Energy. Control the Flow

Money is not merely a financial asset; it reflects focus, discipline, and the exchange of value. It mirrors how you manage your time, energy, and intentions. Just as physical strength requires training and recovery, financial strength demands awareness and structure.

When you view money as energy, you understand it flows where attention and intention go. If you're scattered, reactive, or impulsive, your finances will reflect that instability. If you're deliberate, consistent, and measured, wealth becomes predictable.

Control the flow, or it controls you. A masculine man channels money like power intentionally, efficiently, and with purpose.

Action:

1. Track Every Dollar: Know exactly where your money is going. Daily tracking cultivates discipline and reduces unconscious spending.

2. Set Allocation Rules: Define precise percentages for income for growth, investment, essentials, and reserve. The structure increases control.

3. Remove Emotional Spending: Before making a purchase, pause and ask, "Does this move me forward or distract me from my mission?"

4. Create Systems for Growth: Automate savings, reinvestment, and charitable giving. Energy flows best through systems, not guesswork.

5. Audit Your Circle's Financial Mindset: Align with people who view money as a tool for creation, not just consumption.

Make Bold Decisions, Then Execute Ruthlessly

Masculine power isn't indecision masquerading as strategy; it's clarity transformed into action. The high-level man doesn't wait for the perfect moment; you create it. You see the path, trust your instinct, and move with conviction.

Indecision leaks energy. Overthinking breeds hesitation. Bold decisions backed by ruthless execution set you apart. That's how empires are built, not through luck, but by men who commit fully and follow through, as if their legacy depends on it.

Boldness is not recklessness; it's responsibility in motion. Decide. Move. Adapt. Never stall. The world follows men who walk in conviction.

Action:

1. Decide Within a Time Limit: Give yourself 10 minutes, 10 hours, or 1 day — but set a specific time limit. Bold decisions don't live in procrastination.

2. Cut Plan B: Once committed, remove the escape hatch. Masculine energy sharpens when the mind has no exit, only execution.

3. Schedule Ruthlessly: Put the decision into a time-bound action. Execution lives in the calendar, not in the mind.

4. Eliminate Permission-Seeking: Stop seeking validation. Power is self-sourced. If the decision aligns with your mission, move.

5. Track Results, Not Emotions: Measure your outcomes. Don't get carried away by momentum or bogged down by friction. Stay neutral. Stay precise.

September 8th

Play The Long Game, But Win the Daily

Masculine men think in decades, but they dominate by days. You don't just visualise your empire; you lay bricks every sunrise. The long game is your mission and a legacy you're building to outlive your name. If you don't win the day, the dream stays a fantasy.

The high-level man understands time. You're not in a rush, but you're never idle. You see every choice, workout, call, conversation, breath, as momentum. You don't just show up when it's convenient. You're consistent when it's invisible to others.

Men want greatness without discipline. They crave results without rhythm. The masculine edge requires repetition. Precision. Patience. You don't chase dopamine; you build dopamine from progress. You don't seek comfort; you earn peace through movement.

Long-term vision keeps you sharp. Daily execution keeps you honest, and when those align, people feel it. Business flows more easily, and life respects the man who commits and follows through, not once but again and again.

One day at a time. With relentless presence.

September 9th

Build Leverage Before You Need It

The masculine man doesn't wait for pressure to prepare; he positions early, in the silence before the storm. You don't ask for help when you're desperate. You earn influence while you're calm, sharp, and resourceful.

Leverage is foresight. It's the relationships you've invested in without expecting anything in return. It's the skills you've mastered long before they're required. It's the value you consistently offer, not just when you want something, but because it's who you are.

When you operate like this, pressure doesn't break you; it activates you. Others scramble. You execute. Because you've already built the foundation, and people remember that. They follow the man who thinks ahead. They trust the man who doesn't take but trades value for opportunity, presence for power.

Your dominance becomes undeniable. You don't chase positions. You become the one they call when the room needs strength. When the moment calls for clarity, that's leverage, built by intention, maintained by consistency, and deployed with precision.

Power isn't given. It's stacked. Quietly. Relentlessly. Before the world even knows it's needed.

People Invest in Certainty, Not Ideas

In high-stakes environments, people aren't buying your vision; they're buying you. Not your deck. Not your enthusiasm. Your certainty. Masculine certainty.

Ideas are everywhere. Certainty is rare. It's the energy of a man who's lived it, not just imagined it. Who doesn't flinch when questioned? Who speaks without filler? Who holds eye contact and silence like a weapon.

When you walk into a room with grounded conviction, people feel it. They don't need every detail. They need to know you'll handle it. They know when it hits the wall, you won't collapse; you'll pivot and continue to execute.

Certainty isn't arrogance; it's alignment. Through reps. Through trusting yourself when it would've been easier to fold. That self-trust becomes contagious.

Clients, investors, and partners are not looking for someone who hopes it'll work. They're looking for the man who's already living like it has. That's leadership. That's influence. That's the difference between being heard and being hired.

Negotiate Like a King, Not a Beggar

Negotiation isn't about begging for approval; it's about commanding respect. A masculine man doesn't walk into the room, hoping for a yes. He walks in knowing his value, offering alignment, and setting the tone.

Kings don't plead. They propose. With clarity. With grounded presence. With options, not ultimatums.

When you negotiate from a place of desperation, people smell it. They lowball you. Delay you. Discard you. When you hold your line calm, prepared, and detached from the outcome, the power shifts. You're not chasing the table. You are the table.

This isn't about ego. It's about leverage. It's about knowing what you bring, where you're willing to flex, and where your non-negotiables are. When you negotiate like a king, you teach the world how to treat you, not just in business but in every interaction.

Action:

1. Know your non-negotiables: Write down what you will not compromise on. This is your spine. Don't betray it.

2. Lead with value: Open the conversation by showing how what you offer solves their problem, not yours.

3. Master controlled silence: State your terms. Then wait. No justification. No ramble. Let them respond.

4. Detach from the outcome: Walk away if it's not aligned with your values. Kings don't stay where they're not respected.

5. Follow up with strength: If revisiting the deal, reassert your terms with updated leverage or results.

Attention Is a Currency, Use It, Don't Chase It

Masculine men don't beg for attention. They direct it, and in the high-level game of power, business, and attraction, attention is a form of leverage. The man who chases it becomes reactive, diluted, and forgettable. The man who owns it becomes magnetic. You know that presence creates demand, and demand creates movement.

When you treat attention like currency, you invest it with precision. You decide who gets access when you show up and what message you reinforce. You don't post for likes; you speak for legacy. You don't flood rooms with noise; you enter with weight.

A man of presence doesn't try to be everywhere. He's felt even when he's silent because his name, actions, and presence carry a narrative of value, not validation. You are either a man of attention or a man chasing it. One builds empires. The other gets lost in the noise. Choose the signal. Be the signal.

Action:

1. Audit your output: Where are you spending your attention to gain approval? Cut the noise. Refocus on impact.

2. Speak with intention: Every message, meeting, and action should reinforce who you are and what you stand for.

3. Create demand through absence: Don't be overly accessible. Let your presence feel earned, not taken for granted.

4. Control the narrative: Define the three core traits you want people to associate with you. Ensure every public interaction reflects that.

5. Engage with direction: Don't chase attention. Channel it toward your mission, your vision, and your evolution.

September 13th

Brand Is Reputation at Scale

The brand isn't your logo. It's not your tagline. It's what people say about you when you leave the room, multiplied by every room you'll never be in.

A masculine man understands that his reputation is his authentic brand. It's forged in silence, proven in pressure, and spread through consistency. At the highest levels, in business, leadership, and legacy, your brand becomes your leverage. It's how people decide to trust you, follow you, pay you, or partner with you before they've even met you.

When your brand reflects who you truly are, you don't need to oversell. You don't need to be convinced. Your track record speaks. Your energy confirms it. That's when people start moving in your direction without being asked.

Build a brand rooted in alignment, your values, your discipline, and your integrity. Not hype. Not performance. When the man and the message match, momentum becomes automatic.

The brand is reputation and scaled. You don't chase opportunity. Opportunity recognises you.

September 19th

Watch Body Language, Not Just Words

Words can lie. The body rarely does. A man who understands power reads the unspoken. In business, intimacy, and negotiation, the truth reveals itself in the paused moments, the shift in posture, or the micro-expression, rather than rather than the pitch or the compliment.

Masculine presence sees beyond surface signals. You watch how they breathe, how they blink, how they hold eye contact. You note tension in the jaw, hesitation in the hands, and subtle retreat in their stance.

Gathering intel before you speak is how you lead without being led. Mastering body language makes you more magnetic, more trusted, and more dangerous. You don't just hear what they say, you also see what they do. You feel what they mean.

Master this skill, and you stop chasing validation because you already see the truth before most even sense the tension.

Action: (5–10 mins daily)

1. Choose a setting: a business meeting, a date, or a public setting.

September 14th

Command With Identity

A successful business professional understands that power doesn't come through titles or income; it comes through perception. Your brand is your modern-day coat of arms. A well-forged personal brand is a trust amplifier. When people understand what you stand for and see it reflected in how you move, speak, and deliver, they follow, invest, and align.

For the masculine man, your brand is not fluff. It's a weaponised identity. It tells the world who you are before you open your mouth and sets the terms for how you get paid. Men who operate without a personal brand are constantly chasing relevance. Men who build one are the ones setting direction, commanding deals, and drawing opportunity on their terms. You don't need a million followers. You need a message that is clear and precise and demonstrates value, as evidenced by your results and presence.

Stop selling time and start selling trust to scale your power and business. Your face, your voice, and your presence become the brand, and that's the leverage you own.

Action:

1. Audit your current image across all platforms, including social media, business, and in-person interactions.

2. Do they all align with who you truly are and what you lead in?

3. Cut the noise. Refine your message.

4. Show up daily as the man who already owns what he teaches. Then, let the world catch up.

September 15th

Leadership Is Not Consensus, It's Direction

Masculine leadership isn't about pleasing the room; it's about anchoring it. You were born to chart the path, hold the line, and walk it first.

The man who leads by consensus is fragile. He needs approval before action and validation before voice. Authentic leadership begins with clarity — —a vision so strong that it doesn't shake under pressure. People don't follow uncertainty. They follow the man who moves with certainty, even when it's unpopular.

You don't wait for everyone to agree; you move because it's right. You observe the chaos, listen to the noise, and then make the call that serves the mission, not your ego. Leadership means taking responsibility for outcomes, not just popularity at the moment.

You lead not to control but to direct. Not to be liked but to be trusted. When your decisions consistently create results, people stop questioning your moves. They start aligning with your vision. In a world of indecision and noise, the man who stands firm becomes the compass.

September 16th

Your Calendar Reveals Your Power

Show me your schedule, and I'll show you your standards. A masculine man's calendar isn't complete; it's focused. Every block of time tells a story of priorities, purpose, and precision. You either run your day, or it runs you. The undisciplined man says yes to everything: meetings, favours, distractions. The powerful man protects his time as if his future depends on it because it does.

Your calendar is a mirror of your mission. If it's cluttered with noise, your outcomes will reflect chaos. If it's carved with intention, workouts, strategy, creation, or recovery, you'll move with clarity and force.

Every high-level man knows time is the one resource you never get back. So, your presence, energy, and results begin where your schedule does. Are you investing your time or spending it? Are you building something or reacting to everything? Discipline isn't just about what you do; it's when and how you do it.

Action:

1. Print or screenshot your past 7-day calendar: Highlight what aligned with your goals and what didn't. Be honest.

2. Score each block of time: Rate from 1–10: How much did this task contribute to your long-term vision?

3. Identify and eliminate energy leaks: What calls, meetings, or habits can be eliminated or delegated?

4. Schedule your non-negotiables first: Training. Creation. Strategy. Rest. Lock them in before the noise arrives.

5. Set a weekly review time: Every Sunday or Friday, spend 20 minutes reviewing and planning for the upcoming week. Leadership starts with this ritual.

September 17th

Handle Pressure or Be Handled

Pressure doesn't create the man; it reveals him. In business, in relationships, and in life, pressure is coming. The question is simple: do you collapse, or do you calibrate? A masculine man doesn't avoid tension; you train for it. You see pressure as a forge, not a threat because you know that under load, weakness breaks and strength sharpens.

The man who masters pressure becomes the anchor everyone else leans on. You don't cower when it counts. You hold your edge, keep your breath, and lead with clarity. While others spiral, you remain steady.

Pressure isn't your enemy. It's your proving ground. Handle it or be handled by someone who does.

Action:

1. Expose Yourself to Controlled Stress Daily: Try cold plunges, intense workouts, sparring, or high-stakes calls - choose one. Make discomfort normal.

2. Breathe Under Load: When your heart rate spikes, inhale deeply through your nose and exhale slowly. Regain control, don't react, respond.

3. Simulate High-Stress Scenarios Weekly: Set specific time limits. Add consequences. Rehearse negotiations, sales, public speaking, or decisions under constraints.

4. Debrief the Stress Event: After each pressure moment, review what you did well. What cracked? Where can I tighten?

5. Repeat Under Greater Load: Gradually increase the complexity and stakes. Track how long it takes you to return to a calm, clear state.

September 18th

Study Power Moves in Silence

Absolute power doesn't announce itself. It observes. It calculates. It strikes with precision. The masculine man isn't obsessed with attention; he's obsessed with mastery. While others posture, you study body language, decision-making, negotiation cues, and shifts in hierarchy. You observe how power moves in the room, in deals, and in the relationship dynamics, all without saying a word.

Silence is a strategy that creates space to read the field. It sharpens instincts, and it protects you from playing the fool before you're holding the cards. The men who move the world rarely speak the loudest. They're too busy watching and preparing. When they move, it's surgical. No wasted effort. No scattered energy. It's just pure, directed intent.

2. Scan three people silently: Observe their posture, gestures, and micro-reactions. Are they open or guarded? Confident or compensating? Calm or anxious?

3. Mirror check: Notice your stance. Are you grounded? Chest open? Eyes steady?

4. Apply live: In one conversation, respond not to what they said but to what their body language reveals. Test your reading.

5. Journal your reads: Were you accurate? What did you miss?

Don't Apologise for Taking Up Space

Masculine presence doesn't shrink to make others comfortable. It expands to make others rise. The high-level man knows his worth, and you don't dim it to fit fragile rooms. You walk in with grounded energy, not arrogance. With certainty, not noise. With intent, not permission.

You take up space by the way you breathe, stand, speak with clarity, and act with precision. You don't over-explain. You don't dilute. You don't wait to be chosen because you have already chosen yourself.

Authentic leadership doesn't tiptoe. It stabilises the room simply by arriving, and when you stop apologising for your power, others stop questioning it.

September 21st

Stack Skills Like Weapons

Powerful men aren't born; they purposely and consistently build themselves one sharpened edge at a time. Every skill you develop is a blade in your arsenal—public speaking. Strategic thinking. Emotional control. Negotiation. Discipline. Sales. Storytelling. Leadership. The more you stack, the less you chase. Opportunity flows to the prepared man, not the desperate one.

Masculine growth isn't passive. It's forged. You don't dabble, you dominate. You study, practice, fail forward, and master, then repeat the process. Every room you walk into becomes another arena to test your edge. The weak man relies on one talent and a lucky break. The masculine man becomes a factory for weapons. You evolve in silence and strike with precision when it counts.

Skill stacking creates separation. It turns you into a man of substance, one who's impossible to replace, not because of bravado but because of the results. The future doesn't belong to the strongest. It belongs to the most capable. Build your arsenal. Stay dangerous.

September 22nd

Be Relentlessly Useful

Powerful men don't beg for attention; they command it by being indispensable. In business, in brotherhood, and relationships, the man who solves problems without seeking praise becomes the one everyone turns to when it matters. Being relentlessly practical means, you don't just show up; you upgrade the room, the system, and the energy. It's about being a weapon of service. You bring clarity where there's confusion. direction where there's drift. Calm where there's chaos. You don't waste words, space, or time. You deliver value like it's instinct.

The world isn't waiting for another loud opinion. It's starving for men who can get things done with precision, humility, and edge. Being relentlessly practical makes you unforgettable, not because you talk the most, but because when you're around, everything improves. That's masculine leadership in motion.

Action:

1. 1.Audit Your Strengths: Identify your top three real-world skills. What do you do that makes a difference? Double down.

2. Ask Better Questions: In any room, listen deeply and ask, "What's the biggest leverage problem here I can solve?"

3. Deliver Without Delay: Stop Overthinking. Execute fast. Precision beats perfection.

4. Upgrade Your Tools: Each week, choose one skill to sharpen or one system to streamline. The more efficient you are, the more valuable you become.

5. Leave People Better: Whether it's a conversation, a deal, or a team huddle, always leave them more focused, precise, or empowered.

Success Loves Speed. Don't Wait

Masculine power moves with conviction. It doesn't linger in hesitation, overplanning, or waiting for permission. It scans the terrain, makes the call, and executes. The man who delays under the illusion of perfection will miss opportunities, while the one who moves fast, adjusts on the fly, and learns through action. Speed isn't recklessness; it's decisive momentum. It signals belief. It builds confidence. It separates thinkers from executors.

Every second you hesitate, someone hungrier, more certain, and less attached to being "ready" is making moves you wish you had. That gap becomes your regret. Masculine men don't wait to be perfect; they move with what they've got and build sharper weapons as they go. Speed reveals what planning hides. It opens doors that passive, overthinkers see as locked.

In business, relationships, and personal growth, timing is the hidden king—the man who acts with urgency gains not just progress but presence. You're not reacting. You're responding before most even realise the opportunity was there. When success sees a man in motion, it moves toward him.

September 24th

Audit Who Has Access to You

Masculine presence isn't just about what you give; it's about what you protect. Who gets your time, attention, and energy determines the quality of your focus and outcomes. If you're constantly feeling drained, distracted, or doubting yourself, look at your circle. Access is a privilege, not a right.

High-level men don't allow chaos in the front door and then wonder why their mission derails. They curate who gets proximity because proximity is power. Not everyone deserves to walk with you, especially if they bring confusion, gossip, or stagnation.

Every conversation, every message, every hangout is either sharpening your direction or slowing it down. The man who protects his energy moves faster, clearer, and stronger. Not everyone can go where you're going, and that's precisely how it should be.

Action: (20 Minutes)

1. List the 10 people you interact with most: Friends, clients, family, messages, DMs, all of it.

2. Ask: Does this person energise or drain me? Rate each one: + (adds energy), 0 (neutral), − (drains energy). Be ruthlessly honest.

3. Assess alignment: Does this person align with your mission, values, and future goals? Or are they clinging to your past?

4. Reinforce or reduce: Make bold adjustments —deepen the relationships that build you. Create distance (mentally, emotionally, physically) from those who don't. Set new boundaries where access has been too easy.

5. Lock your gates: Create a new standard: If they don't bring peace, power, or progress, they don't get prime access.

September 25th

Transcend the Boy, Embody the Operator

There's a moment every man faces where excuses, ego, and entitlement no longer suffice. Where seeking validation fades. That's the turning point. That's when the boy falls, and the operator rises.

The boy seeks approval. The operator moves with purpose.
The boy reacts. The operator calculates.
The boy waits for permission. The operator claims space.

Precision replaces overthinking. Discipline replaces doubt. You stop being ruled by your feelings and start being led by your code. The operator doesn't need hype. You're consistent. Strategic. Ruthless with your standards.

Masculine evolution starts when the boy steps aside and the operator steps forward. You don't lose yourself; you finally meet the man you were born to become, with clarity, led by values, and built to execute.

Action:

1. Define your mission: Write down your core purpose. No fluff. What are you here to lead, protect, build, and embody?

2. Audit your softness: Where are you still seeking comfort, avoiding confrontation, or hesitating to take the lead? Name it. That's your edge to sharpen.

3. Discipline one daily habit: Pick the area in which you lack consistency (fitness, food, focus, communication) and dominate it for 30 days. No excuses. No negotiations.

4. Control your inputs: Limit noise. Cut gossip—silence weak opinions. Your focus is your most valuable currency; spend it with intent.

5. Repeat this mantra daily: "I don't need motivation. I move because it's who I am."

September 26th

Strategic Detachment

At a high level, men understand that energy is a form of currency, and where you invest determines your level of power. Emotional overinvestment in people, outcomes, and opinions is how most men drain themselves. It's not love. It's not leadership. It's emotional leakage disguised as care.

Strategic detachment isn't coldness. It's clarity. You can love without clinging. Lead without rescuing. Be present without being pulled under. The person who overinvests emotionally loses control of their time, thoughts, and decisions. You're reactive. You chase closure. You internalise every shift in mood or energy around him.

The masculine man, anchored in detachment, sees the bigger picture. You give but from overflow, not depletion. You hold space but don't abandon yourself in the process. You know when to stay when to let go, and when to reallocate your focus to what moves you forward.

Power isn't in being available to everything. It's in being selective with what owns your mental and emotional bandwidth and where you will spend it.

September 27th

Turn Feedback into Firepower

High-level individuals know that feedback isn't a threat; it's a valuable tool. Used well, it gives you an edge most men avoid. While others defend their ego, you extract data. While they sulk or shrink, you adapt and sharpen.

Feedback shows you where your blind spots lie and where your presence is most effective. Where your results leak, but only if you're grounded enough to hear it without flinching.

Action:

1. Ask the Right People: Don't take opinions from just anyone. Ask trusted allies, mentors, or high-level peers for their input—people who've earned the right to speak about your growth.

2. Separate the Signal from the Emotion: Strip the tone and delivery. Look at what's true in the feedback, not how it made you feel. That's emotional discipline.

3. Extract the Core Truth: Ask: What part of this feedback, if mastered, would move me forward fastest? That's your pressure point. Own it.

4. Build a Response Plan: Write down one habit, system, or behaviour shift you'll apply based on the feedback. Don't wait. Build firepower through action.

5. Close the Loop: After applying the change, review and share the results.

September 28th

Build a Business, Not a Job

If your income stops when you stop, you don't own a business; you own a job. That's a trap most men build with their own two hands. They grind, control every detail, stay busy, and call it entrepreneurship, but the truth is: you didn't escape the 9-5; you just built your cage.

A real business gives you leverage. It works while you sleep. It grows with or without your daily input. It frees your time to think, scale, and lead, and most importantly, it doesn't burn you out. It pays you and gives you peace.

A masculine man builds for freedom, not just profit. He understands that time is the highest currency. You don't win this game by doing more; you win by doing less of what keeps you trapped. Build something that lasts without breaking you.

Action:

1. Audit Your Time: Track your daily tasks for one week. Label each one: $10 task, $100 task, or $10K task. Being buried in low-value tasks creates a bottleneck. Clarity is the first shift.

2. Systemise the Repetitive: Document repeatable tasks and processes. Develop Standard Operating Procedures

(SOPs). To remove your brain from the equation and allow others to step in.

3. Delegate What Drains You: Outsource or hire for the bottom 20% of tasks you're least skilled at or most drained by. Leverage begins when you let go.

4. Productise Your Knowledge: Turn your skills, frameworks, or services into scalable offers, courses, licensing models, group models, and digital products. Your expertise shouldn't need your constant presence.

5. Install Revenue Without You: Build recurring income streams through subscriptions, retainers, and automated funnels. Design at least one channel that generates revenue while you're offline. That's the pivot point.

6. Lead, Don't Just Work: Shift your role from technician to strategist. Start every week with: Where is the business going? What's blocking growth? Who can solve it other than me?

September 29th

Walk Away from Weak Deals Without Flinching

Weak deals aren't always obvious. Sometimes, they are disguised in compliments, urgency, or shiny numbers. They drain more than they deliver. They cost energy, control, reputation, and sometimes, your direction.

The man who knows his worth doesn't bite at every opportunity. You don't say yes out of fear, desperation, or polite obligation. You study the terms, read the energy, and check alignment, not just the upside.

Not every deal that looks "big" is built to last. If it pulls you off the mission, compromises your values, or attaches you to unstable people, it's a weight, not a win. Power isn't in how many deals you close. It's in how many you don't need to.

The masculine man doesn't beg for tables; he builds his own. You're clear on your value, ruthless with your time, and sovereign in your choices. That confidence radiates, and it attracts stronger offers.

You walk away not because you're arrogant but because you're precise. Your mission is too sharp to dilute. Your energy is too valuable to waste, and your legacy is too important to sell at a discount. Say less. Stand tall, and when it's not right, walk. That silence speaks louder than any pitch.

Be the Man Who Doesn't Flinch in the Boardroom

Power in the boardroom doesn't come from how fast you speak, how many slides you prepare, or how big your projections look. It comes from the one thing the masculine man trains relentlessly: inner certainty.

In a room full of egos, projections, and posturing, the man who doesn't flinch becomes the gravity in the room. While others bluff, overcompensate, or scramble for approval, you breathe slower. You speak less, and when you do speak, people listen, not because of volume, but because of weight.

Boardrooms don't reward flash. They reward clarity. The ability to absorb challenge, redirect pressure, and stay grounded when money, reputation, or high-stakes deals are on the line. That's why this isn't about pretending to be confident. It's about becoming the masculine man who's done the reps — physically, mentally, and emotionally — to sit in the pressure cooker without breaking.

Be the one who leans back, not forward. Be the man who doesn't chase agreements but earns them through alignment. Who isn't thrown by interruption, delay, or doubt because you don't walk into that room to prove something? You came to direct the outcome.

This level of masculine presence doesn't just win deals; it builds empires because men who can hold the boardroom steady become trusted not only in business but also in times of crisis. You don't flinch. You command. You lead.

October

Command & Communication

Your voice is your weapon, your shield, your leadership. Use it like one

Your voice is not just sound; it's a signal, and power doesn't come from how loud you speak; it comes from what's behind the words. This month is about mastering your communication like a weapon: clean, calm, and precise. Masculine men don't yell; they speak, and silence follows.

The way you speak is the way you lead. In love, in conflict, in negotiation, or in confrontation, your tone, timing, and presence will either command the room or cost you the outcome. Saying less creates more impact. Speaking with weight and holding a frame with zero emotion, leaking through, and reading the room before owning it.

You'll learn how to lead your woman without controlling her. You'll learn how to speak in rooms where men measure every word. You'll know when to press, when to pause, and when to walk away without saying a thing because your presence has already made the final call.

This month is about unlocking your voice as a force. Not noise. Not ego. Presence. Precision. Pressure.

The man who can command with calm is the man no one wants to go to war with, but everyone wants to stand by.

"Speak with clarity, move with certainty, and be ready for alliance or war; your voice is your weapon."

October 1ˢᵗ

Own Your Tone Before Your Words

A masculine man doesn't speak just to be heard; he speaks to direct, to anchor, to command. Before a single word leaves his lips, his tone has already defined his presence. A room goes quiet, not because a man shouted but because he spoke with stillness. Calm. Controlled cadence. There is no need to fill the space with noise. Just certainty. Just intent.

Your tone tells the world who you are before your message does. It embodies your self-respect, clarity, and emotional mastery. That's why a weak man overtalks, oversells, or seeks approval with every sentence. A masculine man selects words like weapons, few, sharp, and necessary.

When you own your tone, you lead from presence, not pressure. You're not reacting. You're not defending. You're guiding the energy of the room, the conversation, and the outcome.

In negotiation, your tone reveals your edge. In conflict, your tone maintains control. With your woman, your tone either melts her or raises her guard.

It's important to understand that tone is not volume; tone is conviction. It's the grounded energy behind the message that says, "I've already decided who I am."

If you want to lead in war or peace, you must master this first, not just what you say but how you say it. A man who owns his tone owns the moment, and in high-level rooms, that's what turns attention into influence.

October 2ⁿᵈ

Listen With the Intent to Understand, Not to React

Most men listen to the reply. To defend. To fix. The masculine man who has trained his presence listens to understand, and that changes everything. When you truly listen, your eyes stay on hers. Your breath stays calm. Your body stays still. You don't rush to solve, interrupt, or push your point. You receive her fully. That's what makes a woman feel safe, not that you agreed, but that you heard her without judgment.

In leadership, it builds loyalty. In conflict, it defuses tension. In intimacy, it opens doors that words alone can't. Masculine communication isn't always about having the best words; it's about conveying the right message. It's about having the strongest space, the kind of space where others can show up fully and feel seen in it. When you lead with presence, watch how connection, respect, and influence multiply.

Action:

1. Pause Before You Respond: Count silently to 3 after they finish speaking. It creates space and prevents emotional reactions.

2. Mirror the Message: Briefly repeat what they said in your own words. Example: "So what I hear you saying is…"

3. Ask, Don't Assume: Use one follow-up question to dig deeper. "What made you feel that way?" or "What's most important to you about this?"

4. Hold Your Frame: Don't rush to fix or agree. Stay calm. Let your presence communicate strength, not noise.

5. Reflect Alone: After the conversation, write down one thing you learned about the person, not the topic, to train deeper awareness.

October 3rd

Listen With the Intent to Understand, Not to React

Masculine presence doesn't rush to fix, defend, or explain. It absorbs. When you listen not to respond but to understand, you disarm chaos, deepen trust, and command the moment.

In a world obsessed with being heard, true power is being the man who hears everything: tone, breath, silence, and subtext. That's the kind of man women lean into, and teams align with and stand behind. Not because you talk the most but because when you do speak, your words cut through the noise.

When you choose to understand before reacting, your words land sharply. Your leadership holds more weight. Your relationship becomes safer, and your presence becomes magnetic. You're not just hearing people. You're seeing them, and in a reactive world, that's a rare occurrence.

Master the silence.

October 4th

Say Less, Mean More

In high-stakes rooms, relationships, and leadership, words are currency. The more you speak, the more you risk deflating your value, but the man who speaks with precision becomes unforgettable.

When you say less, but every word carries weight, people lean in. Your woman trusts your leadership. Your team listens, and your clients believe because you've trained yourself to speak only when it matters and when you do, it's with clarity, not just noise.

You don't chase validation through volume. You don't fill silence with small talk. You hold space, and you communicate with your eyes, your breath, and your tone long before the words come.

In a world addicted to overexplaining and over-posting, be the man who moves with measured conviction. That's not silence out of fear; that's presence forged in confidence.

Masculine men don't talk to be heard.

October 5th

Your Presence Speaks First, Master It

Before you say a word, your presence announces you. Not your outfit, not your business card, your energy. The masculine man doesn't need to perform. He stands still, and people notice. He looks, and people pay attention. He speaks, and people lean in because they feel him first.

Presence is trained in your posture, breath, eye contact, and your ability to hold tension without needing to release it. It's in how grounded you are in your values. How certain you are in your direction. How little do you need to prove?

Presence isn't just for public moments; it's forged in private discipline. In how you carry yourself at the gym. In how you listen to your woman. In how you lead when no one's clapping.

Masculine presence is calm, not chaotic. It's stable, not stiff. It's the quiet force that shifts the atmosphere without force. You don't demand attention; you earn it by how well you embody yourself. Be the man who walks in fully arrived, and your energy is the loudest thing in the room.

October 6th

Speak Like a Weapon

A powerful man doesn't raise his voice; he sharpens it. Your words are few, but every word has clarity, conviction, and control. That's the difference between speaking and commanding.

When you speak like a weapon, you cut through the noise. You don't fluff. You don't over-explain. You don't defend your value; you embody it. Masculine speech isn't aggressive; it's precise. It moves people because it's rooted in certainty, not emotion.

You don't just say what's popular. You say what's needed, even if it's uncomfortable. Especially then because men of impact know the truth is rarely loud, but it's always sharp.

This style of speech doesn't come from memorising scripts. It comes from knowing who you are, where you stand, and what you'll never tolerate. That inner alignment gives your words force.

October 7th

Know When to Interrupt and When to Let Silence Work

Interrupting isn't always disrespectful; it's a strategy. A high-level man knows when a moment needs redirection, a truth inserted, or a boundary drawn. He also knows the greater weapon is silence.

Silence creates tension. Space. Power. It allows truth to land. It reveals who's uncomfortable, and it forces others to lean in. Weak men rush to fill gaps. Masculine men know those gaps are leverage. You don't speak to kill time; you talk to command it.

Interrupt when the moment is going off-track, when someone needs protection, or when a boundary is being tested. Hold the silence when the room is full of noise, emotion is high, or truth is about to echo because real power isn't always in what you say; it's in what you're unshaken enough to leave unsaid.

October 8th

Communicate Through Energy, Not Volume

Masculine communication is precise. You speak with energy that carries weight, and people feel it before they even hear it. You don't force attention. You direct it.

Raising your volume often reveals insecurity. Controlled energy reveals certainty. When you own your body, your breath, and your intent, every word lands with impact. That's how masculine men speak from the gut, not the throat.

Your tone should match your mission:

- Calm when others panic.
- Direct when others dodge.
- Grounded when others grasp.

People don't remember the pitch. They recognise the presence.

Action:

1. Master your breath: Speak on the exhale. It keeps you calm and grounded.

2. Pause before you speak: This adds authority. Rushed men aren't trusted.

3. Drop your tone: A lower vocal register conveys power. Not aggression or control.

4. Use stillness: Avoid fidgeting or over-gesticulating. Your stillness says, "I'm in charge."

5. Make eye contact, then speak: Let your energy arrive first. Your words will follow with more force.

October 9th

Look People in the Eye Until They Shift

When a man locks eyes, not to intimidate, but to witness, it changes the dynamic. In leadership, relationships, and negotiations, eye contact is a key aspect that is often made visible. It tells the other person: I'm here, I see you, I won't break.

Most people look away when it gets real. Masculine men lean in. You're not starting to dominate. You're holding space. That still gaze says more than noise ever could. It earns trust in seconds. It shows you're unshaken, and when you don't flinch, they're the one who shifts.

Whether you're speaking to a woman, an investor, or your reflection, eye contact reveals who trusts themselves and who's bluffing. Masculine presence is felt and seen. Your eyes are the proof.

Action:

1. Hold gaze during every greeting: Don't rush the handshake or break eye contact. Anchor it.

2. Practice silent connection: With a partner or friend, sit in silence for 60 seconds and maintain eye contact. Notice your reactions.

3. Speak your truth while looking them directly in the eye, especially when it's uncomfortable. Truth needs a spine.

4. Don't scan the room: own the space, whether in meetings or on a date and lock into one set of eyes at a time. Make people feel chosen.

5. Use your eyes to calm, not cut: Soften the aggression. Replace it with an unshakable presence.

October 10th

Master the Art of Saying No

Weak men overcommit. They seek approval, avoid conflict, and dilute their power with scattered energy. Masculine men draw precise lines. They know that every time you say "yes" to something misaligned, you're saying "no" to your mission.

Your time, attention, and energy are finite; treat them like a sovereign asset. "No" isn't rude. It's refined. It's how kings move. When you can decline offers, invites, distractions, and even people without guilt, you step into true command. You stop reacting to the world and start shaping it.

Saying "no" is presence. It's direction. It's a declaration: I don't owe you access to my time; I own it. You don't need to be aggressive. You need to be grounded. A man who can say "no" with calm certainty owns the room and his life.

Action:

1. Audit your last 10 commitments: Which ones drained your energy? Which moved you closer to your goals? Cut the first.

2. Use the 3-second rule: When asked for your time, pause for 3 seconds. Breathe. If it's not a clear yes, it's a no.

3. Stop explaining your boundaries: "No" is a complete sentence. Let silence reinforce it.

4. Rehearse in front of a mirror: Say no with eye contact, relaxed body language, and a grounded tone. Train your nervous system to stay focused and alert.

5. Honour your 'no' like a contract: Every time you fold, you fracture self-trust. Stay firm. Stay free.

October 11th

Don't Flinch in Conflict, Hold Frame

Anyone can speak well when the room is calm, but when tension rises, voices rise, and egos swell, the real test begins.

High-level men don't chase dominance through aggression. They hold the frame. That means staying calm when challenged and measured when provoked. Clear when others scramble. Holding the frame is about being the gravity in the room, not the storm.

When you hold your frame, you don't just win the moment; you influence the energy of the room. You become the thermostat, not the thermometer. Conflict doesn't unnerve you; it sharpens you, and that's precisely why people follow your lead.

Action:

1. Train your body under pressure: cold plunges, combat drills, and high-stakes decision-making. Get familiar with discomfort.
2. Slow your breath before you speak: In conflict, your breath controls your mind. Inhale for 4, exhale for 6.
3. Ground your posture: Shoulders back, jaw relaxed, feet solid. Don't posture. Don't shrink. Stay rooted.

4. Say less, watch more: Use silence as a weapon. Let others react while you observe patterns.

5. Pre-frame your standards: Let people know who you are and what you don't tolerate before conflict arises. That's real power.

October 12th

Words Mean Nothing Without Backing

In the world of high-level men, nobody cares what you say; they care what you prove. You can speak of values, vision, and intent all day, but without aligned action, it's noise. Masculine communication isn't measured in syllables; it's in the outcome.

The man who says little but moves heavily is always respected more than the man who says everything but delivers nothing. Power isn't in how loudly you talk; it's in the consistency behind the talk. Backing your words turns language into leverage.

In every room, boardroom, bedroom, and battlefield, men are silently calculating: Can I trust what he just said? Will he follow through? If the answer is yes, your word becomes law. If not, you lose the room before you even start.

Action:

1. Audit your talk-to-action ratio: How often do you say things you don't do? Eliminate even the smallest false promises.

2. Make fewer commitments but go all in on each: Overpromising weakens trust. Under-promise and over-execute.

3. Align speech with reputation: If you want to be seen as a man of action, let your calendar and results do the talking.

4. When you say it, own it: Your name represents every commitment. Follow through as if it's a legacy because it's.

October 13th

Speak to the Truth, Not the Emotion

When tension rises, weak men yield to their emotions. Strong men anchor to the truth. In conversations, especially with emotionally charged partners, employees, or friends, the masculine man listens fully but doesn't get swept up in the storm.

You see the feeling but speak to the fact. That's not cold. That's clarity, and clarity is what brings resolution, not reaction.

Masculine communication means not escalating emotions and avoiding invalidating them. You acknowledge it and then guide the conversation back to reality, direction, and outcome. You lead through the fog. When everyone else is emotional, the man who can stay centred and speak what's real becomes the anchor others trust.

Action:

1. Pause before speaking: When emotion rises, breathe. Ground yourself before you respond.
2. Validate the feeling, but steer toward the truth: Say, "I get that you're upset," then follow it with, "Let's look at what happened."

3. Ask truth-revealing questions: Use clarity drivers, such as "What do we both agree on?" or "What changed?"

4. Use a neutral, weighty tone: Speak in a low, slow, and confident tone—your tone calms before your words land.

5. Refuse to be pulled into drama: If it spirals, hold your ground: "I'm here for the truth, not to trade reactions."

October 14th

Know the Difference Between Influence and Control

Masculine presence isn't about bending the world to your will; it's about moving through it with such clarity and weight that others want to align with you. That's influence.

Control, on the other hand, is a form of force. It's fear in disguise. It demands, coerces, and micromanages, and it always fractures relationships, trust, and leadership.

Influence is quiet power; it speaks with conviction, acts with integrity, and respects free will. It doesn't chase. It doesn't beg. It simply becomes so grounded in truth that people adjust around it.

Control is reactive. Influence is grounded, and the high-level masculine man knows that trying to control a woman, a team, or a situation is a weakness wearing dominance. You don't seek obedience; you create alignment. The more aligned you are within, the less you need to force anything externally.

True power doesn't dominate. It inspires. It elevates, and it moves without resistance because the world follows the man who's already sure of himself.

October 15th

Give Her Direction,
Not Dominance

A high-level, masculine man doesn't bark orders. He doesn't manipulate. He doesn't lead from insecurity masked as control. You hold a vision. You have clarity, and you invite your woman into it with presence, not pressure.

Dominance demands submission.

Direction creates safety.

Dominance is about power over.

Direction is about power.

When you lead with direction, she feels considered, not commanded. She softens because she knows you see the whole board, not just your ego. She surrenders because she wants to, not because she must. That's where the polarity comes alive when your grounded leadership gives her space to flow fully into her feminine.

If you're forcing it, you've already lost her. The true masculine direction doesn't shrink her; it expands her. It sets the pace. It builds the path, and it trusts her to walk it beside you, not behind you.

October 16th

Don't Be Afraid to Let Her Walk

When you fear her leaving, you stop leading. You start negotiating your integrity. You start softening your standards. You start over-explaining, over-accommodating, and over-apologising.

That's not love; that's fear dressed in need, and a man in his masculine knows that genuine connection can't be forced or begged for. If you've shown up with presence, strength, and integrity, and she still chooses to leave, let her.

What stays out of fear drains you.

What stays out of respect fuels you.

What comes back without force is real.

You don't need to prove your worth by holding tighter. You prove it by letting go when it no longer aligns with your values. The man who's not afraid to lose her becomes the man she respects, even if she walks.

October 17th

Power Moves Require Calm Execution

Power isn't frantic. It's not reactive. It's precise. When making high-stakes decisions, whether in business, conflict, or relationships, your calm is your leverage. As a masculine man, you don't announce your plans. You read the field, sharpen your strike, and execute without emotion clouding the move. Emotion is noise. Calm is clarity.

There's nothing more commanding than a man who acts without flinch and fanfare. No need to posture. No need to warn. It's just a decision made with full presence, followed by execution that doesn't miss.

That's what separates operators from amateurs; when you can move calmly under fire, you don't just look powerful —you are powerful. That's when doors open, respect sharpens, and outcomes shift in your favour. Silence the noise. Then strike.

October 18th

Speak to Her Safety, Not Her Ego

Masculine communication in relationships isn't about charming your way into her attention. It's about anchoring her in certainty, both emotionally and physically, and energetically. Women remember how you made them feel. Not the compliments, but the calm. Not the lines but the presence behind your words.

Her ego might enjoy flattery, but her body and spirit crave safety. When a woman feels safe, she opens up. She softens. She surrenders emotionally, mentally, and sexually. That only happens when your words, tone, body language, and leadership convey security, not performance.

If you're chasing approval, trying to impress, or manipulating through words, she'll feel it and withdraw.

Action:

1. Regulate your energy first: Before speaking, breathe deeply and ground yourself in your body. Your calm becomes a signal.

2. Lower your voice and pace: Speak more slowly. Deeper. From your diaphragm. Women feel tonal vibration more than content.

3. Hold eye contact, but don't chase it: Look at her, not through her. Let your presence say, "I see you, and I'm not leaving."

4. Speak truth, not flattery: Tell her what's real. "I notice you've been carrying a lot. You don't have to with me." That's safety. That's leadership.

5. Frame the future with direction, not doubt: "Here's what I'm building. You're part of it, not just today, but when things get heavy too." That speaks to her heart, not just her edges.

October 19th

Arguments Are a Weak Men's Sport

Arguments are noise. They're a sign that you have lost your sense of perspective, are experiencing emotional instability, or need to prove something. Masculine men don't play that game. They don't wrestle for dominance through raised voices or scattered emotion because they know the louder the voice, the weaker the stance.

You don't need to win a shouting match when your presence says more than your words ever could. You don't need to defend your worth when it's already felt. Strong men speak once and move accordingly.

When a masculine man is challenged, he listens. Not to react but to read the room. You know what's yours and what's hers. What's worth addressing, and what's a test of your poise? That's when you hold your centre and let others spin if they choose to. You don't chase the chaos.

Arguments pull you into her emotion, her storm, her test. When you get pulled, you fail the test. The masculine man stays grounded. He speaks to the truth, not tantrums. You navigate tension like a compass, not a weapon. You don't raise your voice; you lower the room's tension with your calm voice. You take the lead, even in conflict.

Leadership in love isn't proven when things are good. It's proven when things are heated, and you remain unshaken.

Remember: the moment you argue, you give away your position. The moment you anchor, you keep your power. Masculine men don't argue; they execute.

October 20th

Let Silence Expose the Truth

In a world addicted to noise, silence is a powerful force. It disarms. It reveals. It separates the grounded from the reactive. The man who can sit in silence without fidgeting, without explaining, without needing to fill the gap owns the frame.

Most people speak to cover their insecurity. To fill space. To buy time. When you stop talking, you start seeing. You see the flinch. The contradiction. The bluff. You see whether her words match her body. Whether a man is bluffing or certain. Whether the energy in the room shifts or steadies.

Silence forces truth to rise. It makes liars uncomfortable, and the insecure tend to overexplain.

It allows a woman to reveal her actual needs without you having to pry.

Masculine men use silence like a scalpel, precise, intentional, surgical. They don't rush to respond. They let the weight of their presence create space where truth can't hide.

You don't intimidate with volume. You dominate with stillness. Let others fill the space. Let them reveal their hand. You already know yours. Let silence expose the game, the story, and the truth. When you do speak, do it with clarity, not emotion.

October 21st

In Business, Every Word is a Lever

In high-level business, words are not fillers; they're force. Each sentence you speak either elevates your position or exposes your lack of precision. Every pitch, every answer, every response is a lever: it either moves people closer to trust or pushes them further into doubt.

Overexplaining signals insecurity. Vagueness kills deals.

The masculine communicator speaks with weight. You understand tone, timing, and tempo. You don't "sell" your position. You don't talk in circles; you drop weighted words, then let that point sit. When you speak, people lean in because it's clear you're not trying to impress; you're moving something.

A word can trigger urgency. A phrase can shift perception. A sentence can lead to investment. That's the art of verbal leverage. Whether you're negotiating contracts, leading a team, or building a brand, the wrong words dilute your value the same way too many words do. The right ones expand it. High-value men train this like a weapon.

You pause before you speak.

You use silence as your punctuation.

You don't promise, you state.

You don't convince, you confirm.

In business, your words are not just sounds; they're strategy, and when your words have hit and the outcome solid, you wrap up the conversation and leave. You create momentum, reinforce credibility, and anchor your presence in the room long after you've left it.

Every word you say either moves money, power, or people. Speak like you know that.

October 22nd

Confront Without Emotion, That's Power

In high-stakes environments, such as business, relationships, and leadership, confrontation is not a sign of weakness. It's a necessity. How you confront defines whether you lead or lose.

The immature man reacts. His tone spikes. His ego flares. His need to be right overrides his need to be effective. The masculine man confronts with clarity. You bring the facts, not the fury. You don't posture or provoke; you position with control, moving the outcome your way.

Confrontation without emotion is control. It's your edge without chaos. It's the steel in your spine and the stillness in your tone. You're not avoiding the issue; you're containing it, directing it, and leading it.

The man who can look another man in the eye, call the truth out and hold the line without raising his voice is the untouchable man.

October 23rd

Learn to De-Escalate Like a King

De-escalation is not a weakness. It's mastery. When tension rises, egos flare, and energy spikes, the average man reacts. The king recalibrates. You don't match chaos with chaos. You contain, observe and command it.

This isn't passive. This is precision. You don't back down. You slow down. You lower your tone, not your power. You read the room, not react to it. You listen to the noise with precision to know what each person's needs are behind all the bravado, and then you choose your words with depth and weight that brings order.

Kings don't brawl; they build order. They don't lose their edge just because someone else lost theirs.

To de-escalate like a king means:

- You pause when others panic
- You speak when silence cuts deeper
- You lock in when others lash out

You understand that presence beats volume. Stillness beats shouting, and strategy beats reaction every time.

October 24th

Speak Your Standards, Not Your Insecurities

Masculine men don't need to over-explain, justify, or overcompensate. They don't bark their value or demand respect; they hold a standard, and they speak it with clarity.

When an insecure man speaks, his tone becomes defensive; he seeks validation, tries to convince, or asks for permission.

When you speak from your standard, your presence speaks first. You state what you allow, what you won't tolerate, and what you expect, not to dominate but to align. There's no emotion behind it. It's just conviction, not convincing.

When your voice aligns with your values, the world adjusts.

Action:

1. Audit Your Language: Record or write down how you communicate in moments of tension. Are you reacting? Justifying? Seeking to be liked?

2. Clarify Your 3 Non-Negotiables: Define your standards in relationships, business, and self. Keep them short, clear, and firm. E.g., "I don't explain twice. I lead once."

3. Practice Calm Assertion: Say your standard aloud in a neutral tone. No aggression. No apology.

4. Catch the Insecurity Before It Speaks: Before you speak in a high-stakes moment, pause. Ask: "Am I speaking to be heard or speaking to be validated?"

5. Anchor in Your Body: Breathe deeply, feel your feet on the ground, and speak slowly. Presence is power; it keeps your standard clear and your message sharp.

October 25th

Know When to End the Conversation

A masculine man knows when a conversation has served its purpose. You don't argue in circles. You don't beg to be understood. You don't stay in a space where clarity is no longer being built but is breaking.

Words have weight and wasting them weakens your presence. If your point has value and weight, and the other side is still spiralling in reaction, drama, or disrespect, you don't need to keep talking. You exit with poise, not pettiness.

Control isn't about dominating the last word. It's about knowing you've already said the words that matter. When you can walk away with your energy intact, your standard upheld, and your mind clear, you've already won, and the conversations don't linger in your mind of what you could've or should've said. It's done

October 26th

Raise Your Standards, Not Your Voice

Power isn't about volume; it's about value. When a man knows what he stands for in relationships, business, and life, he doesn't need to argue or overexplain his position. He holds the line.

Raising your voice is a reaction.

Raising your standard is a decision.

It means you no longer tolerate chaos, excuses, disrespect, or energy that drags you below your purpose. You don't plead for better; you require it by how you move, speak, and the choices you make.

In leadership, it means setting clear expectations and letting actions back them. In love, it means honouring your values and walking if they're compromised. In self-mastery, it means not letting your feelings lower your frequency.

Others will test your edges. They'll try to pull you into emotional noise, bait you into defence, or distract you from your frame. Read them and their intentions, then hold your ground in silence and strength, and take a few calming breaths because real power doesn't react; it chooses. When you speak less and align more, your silence becomes sharper than any shout.

October 27th

In Every Interaction: Ally, Exit, or War

Every person you meet is one of three things: An Ally. Dead Weight. Or A Threat.

High-level men don't waste energy wondering. They observe patterns, read energy, and quickly sort people. You become efficient in time, energy output, or resources.

Ally means they elevate you. They match your standards. They challenge you to grow, not shrink. You collaborate, build, and exchange value. Keep these close. Feed the bond.

Deadweight means they aren't aligned, not good, not bad, just not it: misaligned energy, mismatched values, or dead conversations. Don't force. Don't fix it. Exit clean.

War doesn't mean drama; it implies resistance. Opposition. If someone's trying to manipulate, undermine, or control you, you don't flinch. You don't fight emotionally. You outthink, outpace, outlast. Calm dominance.

Action: The 3-Second Sort
Next time you're in a conversation, personal or professional, ask yourself:

1. Does this person add value or drain it?
2. Are they walking alongside you or slowing your pace?
3. If things got difficult, would they stand by you or turn against you?

   If the answer is "ally," decide on concrete values and benefits moving forward.

   If it's "dead weight," exit.

   If it's "war," plan your next move.

   Masculine power isn't about playing every game. It's about knowing which arena you belong in and who's worth entering it with.

October 28th

Set Boundaries with Your Voice, Not Your Fists

For the masculine man, strength isn't just physical; it encompasses energy, psychology, and vocal expression. When you honour a boundary with calm certainty, people feel it in their nervous system. Your voice becomes the perimeter of your values. Not loud. Not reactive. Just final.

Weak men escalate, shout, deflect, attempt to discredit you or lash out when they feel disrespected. Because they haven't developed genuine inner strength. The masculine man doesn't need to prove his capability. Your tone is measured, your presence steady, and your words hold depth: restraint grounded in strength.

You're capable of violence. You've trained for it, you know your edge, and you know what you're capable of if the situation demands it. That's precisely why you don't need to show it. You choose peace over war. It's an unspoken presence that other men feel in the room. They see it in how you carry yourself —relaxed, controlled, yet unmistakably dangerous if crossed. That presence alone keeps the wrong ones in check without a word and the right men with mutual respect.

Setting boundaries with your voice isn't about weakness; it's the ultimate display of discipline. You don't need fists when your conviction is already louder than any threat. Speak once. Speak clearly. Let the stillness behind your words carry the weight of your potential.

Action:

1. Recall a moment where you allowed disrespect to pass unchecked.
2. Revisit it. Ask yourself: Did I speak with finality? Did my tone reflect my standards?
3. Practice that tone now: controlled, grounded, unapologetic.
4. Let every word from here forward reflect the man who chooses power over noise, command over chaos.

October 29th

Speak in Facts, Not Feelings

In high-level environments, business, leadership, and relationships, it's not the loudest voice that commands attention. It's the clearest. The man who speaks facts doesn't get pulled into drama. You don't argue with subjective emotions. You anchor your words and the moment in truth.

Here's the difference:

Feelings say, "You never listen to me."

Facts say, "I spoke for 3 minutes, and you interrupted twice."

Feelings say, "This deal feels wrong."

Facts say, "The ROI projections dropped 18% from last quarter."

When you speak from emotion alone, you invite opinion. Debate. Weak rebuttal.

If you talk from grounded facts, you cut through the mud.

Masculine men don't suppress emotions; you have a trained, self-aware relationship with them. You process your feelings before you speak. You clarify internally, then deliver externally. That's how you stay powerful in conversations, even heated ones. You don't lose the frame. You breathe, recalibrate when needed, and you deliver with clarity.

You don't need to be robotic. You need to be grounded. Feelings are fuel, and facts are the map.

When your truth is clean, your leadership becomes undeniable.

October 30th

Be Unshakeable in the Face of Manipulation

Manipulation is emotional warfare. It's subtle. It's disguised as guilt, flattery, gaslighting, or playing the victim. It only works on the man who hasn't mastered himself.

When someone attempts to control you through emotion, the weak person often reacts by defending, over-explaining, or giving in to keep the peace. The masculine man sees the pattern. You hold your ground. You don't raise your voice. You don't try to win the moment. You let the truth sit in the room, and you don't move. When you're grounded, manipulation becomes obvious and powerless.

Action:

1. Recalibrate Your Nervous System: When you feel your body getting tight or triggered, don't speak yet. Breathe. Slow. Nose in, mouth out. Get back in your body.

2. Call Out the Pattern, Not the Person: Say calmly, "That feels like an emotional tactic. Let's stay focused on what's real." Or: "I'm not available for guilt games. Let's talk directly."

3. Hold Your Tone: Don't match their chaos. Lower your tone. Shorten your words. When your energy is calm and immovable, theirs either shifts or exposes itself.

4. Set a Clear Boundary: "If we can't speak in clarity and honesty, I'll step away until we can." Boundaries are not threats. They're standards.

5. Reflect Later, Not During: Post-conversation, ask yourself:

    o   What did they want from me?
    o   What tactic was used?
    Did I hold my line with honour?

October 31st

Truth Over Tension

A masculine man doesn't shy away from hard conversations. You don't hide behind silence, fake peace, or passive behaviour to keep things comfortable. You speak the truth, even when the room is tight. Tension is not the enemy. It's the threshold.

Every breakthrough in life, love, business, or brotherhood is on the other side of a moment where most men shrink. They swallow their truth to avoid being disliked, misunderstood, or abandoned. When you walk in truth, tension becomes a tool, not a threat. It sharpens clarity. It reveals character and clears up the confusion.

The masculine man speaks clearly and directly, never cutting but rather clarifying. You don't lash out, manipulate, or sugarcoat the truth. You deliver your message with a grounded tone, maintaining eye contact and conveying purpose.

Truth, when delivered with presence, doesn't push people away. It draws the right people closer and filters the rest, building trust and leadership.

Your legacy is anchored in the strength of voice control and command.

If you want to be respected, stop hiding what you know needs to be said. Have hard conversations face-to-face. Not with aggression. Not with emotion but with calm certainty.

That's the masculine edge.

Pushing Limits

Expand Your Edges. Seek Discomfort. Embrace Challenge. Thrive Under Pressure

Everything you want lives past the edge you're currently standing on. This month isn't about motivation; it's about confrontation. With your limits. Your laziness. Your excuses. Masculine men grow through pressure, not comfort, and this is where you stop avoiding challenges and start demanding them.

You're not here to stay safe; you're here to get sharper, more complex, and more dangerous by choice. Discomfort is the test. Pain is the feedback. The challenge is the gift. Every time you step into something that challenges your mind, body, and emotions; you expand. That's the masculine path. Relentless, strategic, and savage when needed.

This month, you will seek resistance and make it your training ground. You'll step into uncertainty and lead anyway. You'll break the habit of backing away, delaying, or being half-committed, and you'll start rising through deliberate pressure. The man who trains to thrive in chaos is the one who dominates when the moment calls.

"A man doesn't grow by surviving; he evolves by stepping into the unknown by choice."

November 1st

Choose the Hard Path on Purpose

The easy path has never built greatness, and the masculine man knows it. When you deliberately choose the more challenging route, you sharpen and strengthen the weapon that is yourself.

This path is intentional. It's choosing to train when it's cold and dark outside. It's choosing to remove pleasures to stay on your mission. It's walking alone through the fire, knowing your purpose calls you. It's speaking the uncomfortable truth when silence would be easier. It's taking on the high-stakes mission that others step away from because your identity grounds in facing adversity head-on.

By walking the hard road on purpose, you train your nervous system to regulate under pressure. While weaker men panic, flee, or collapse. You breathe deeper and move smoothly, building internal armour that is subtle but powerful.

The masculine man becomes efficient in high stakes, high-pressure and high-risk moments. You stop reacting and start refining. Every challenge you walk into on your terms strengthens a layer of your psyche that cannot be shaken. You earn an unspoken edge, presence without words, dominance without threat, trust without explanation.

Building mental toughness, precision, and conditioning shape you for life's hard hits later when you don't see them coming to carve out your leadership.

Action:

1. Pick one area where you've defaulted to comfort, something small but symbolic.
2. Flip it: Choose the more challenging route today, not to suffer, but to sharpen your skills.
3. Train your breath through it.
4. Notice how your mind fights and command it to strengthen you.

Get Comfortable Being Uncomfortable

Discomfort is not your enemy. It's your gateway. It's the pressure point that separates men who fold from men who move forward. The average man avoids it, numbing out, chasing comfort, or overreacting as if they're under attack. The masculine man leans in. You see discomfort not as something to escape but as something to master.

Discomfort is the training ground. It's the mirror that shows you exactly where you're soft, undisciplined, or disconnected. Your breath shortens—your body tenses. Your mind starts hunting for exits. Good. That's where the work begins.

It's not about suffering for the sake of suffering; it's about full-spectrum awareness by choosing to face the physical, mental, and emotional tension head-on and refusing to flinch. That kind of presence makes you dangerous in the best way. In business, you don't break under pressure; you get sharper. In relationships, you don't pull away in silence; you stay with the weight of your truth. In life, when chaos hits, you're already grounded.

While others run from discomfort, you become fluent in it. You learn to breathe calmly and deeply in the tension. You stop looking for comfort as a reward and start using resistance as your compass. Discomfort reveals where the breakthrough lies.

When you choose to stay calm in discomfort, you build a level of undeniable internal strength. You walk into rooms with gravity. You hold presence under pressure. You become the man others turn to when it all goes sideways, not because you talk the loudest, but because you've trained where they've tapped out, and in the chaos, you've learnt to dominate.

Action:

1. Find your edge physically, emotionally, or mentally and go there on purpose.
2. Hold the position: Sit in the tension. Don't escape. Don't numb. Breathe.
3. Observe: Let discomfort reveal what you need to strengthen.

Do One Thing Daily That Scares You

Fear isn't your enemy; it's your frontier. It points to where you stop and where you grow. For the masculine man, that's precisely where your work begins.

The modern world has created men who crave certainty, who numb their instincts with comfort, and who calculate every move before taking it. That's not power. That's stagnant paralysis.

True power expands by choice, not by chance. When you deliberately move toward what you fear the most, you break the illusion that it owns you, and you release the pressure it holds on to you. You stop waiting for life to test you and begin testing yourself, shifting from a reactive to a proactive mindset without fear but with clarity.

Not every test needs to be extreme. What matters is that it's real with an unknown outcome. Every time you confront that edge, your nervous system adapts. Your mind sharpens. Your self-trust deepens. Facing fear daily doesn't make you fearless; it makes you ready.

Action:

1. Identify Today's Edge: What scares you today? Is it a conversation you've been avoiding? A cold plunge? A business risk? A moment of real emotional vulnerability?

2. Approach It Consciously: Don't rush. Don't overthink. Breathe. Feel the fear. Then, walk into it calmly and with full awareness.

3. Complete It Fully: No half-steps. If you step in, finish the move. Own it. If you fall short, don't retreat; adapt and figure it out to get it done.

4. Process Immediately After: Write down what you felt before, during, and after and how you got through it.

5. Capture the moment: Take an intentional breath once you've conquered the fear to anchor it in your nervous system

Pursue the Challenge, Not the Reward

A man who chases the climb, who seeks the test and the unknown, becomes something different. You become unshakable.

Don't be addicted to applause, milestones, and the dopamine of winning.

When you stop obsessing over what you'll get and start focusing on who you'll become through the pursuit itself, you enter a different league. That's when discipline becomes a joy. Reps become ritual. The path becomes who you are.

It's not that you don't want results; it's that they no longer define you. Whether you win or lose, the real prize is the man you become because of the path you choose. You don't question your purpose when the reward isn't immediate. You don't compromise when it gets hard, confusing, or lonely. You stay the course because the course is the sharpening stone for you, your purpose, and your legacy.

Outcomes fade. Accolades are forgotten. The man who has stepped into tests walks courageously. That's what makes you unstoppable.

November 5th

Delay Gratification, Stretch the Tension

Masculine power isn't built in the sprint through life, collecting trophies to announce. It comes from the long path, the one full of milestones hit in silence, internal victories claimed without applause. It's the man who sees the next achievement coming, feels the hunger rise in his gut, then calmly breathes, captures the moment, and moves forward. There is no need to broadcast. No need to break stride. Just progress. Quiet. Focused. Unstoppable.

Delayed gratification is a discipline in motion. It's the art of holding the energy instead of leaking it for a quick dopamine hit. The longer you can stretch the tension, the more force you can build behind your next move.

When you delay pleasure, you sharpen precision. You don't overreach in business; you time your moves like a tactician. You don't fumble in relationships; you stay grounded in presence. In sex, you don't collapse under impulse; you extend the connection, own the space, and lead with depth. That restraint amplifies your power, giving you the ability to command your energy rather than be owned by it.

Separating the kings from the restless boys. You don't chase the crown; you earn it, one step at a time. Every breath between the milestones resets your clarity. Every moment you resist the urge to celebrate too early, you sharpen your mission. When the time finally comes to strike, to claim, to build, to conquer, you do it from a place of focused intention.

Action:

1. Choose one area of your life, training, sex, food, business, or validation, and stretch the tension.
2. Delay the reward.
3. Breathe deeper when the urge rises.
4. Hold it. Own it.
5. Redirect that energy into your pursuit.
6. Keep going. The man who delays gratification moves faster because you aren't chasing; you're building.

November 6th

Finish What You Start

Masculine strength isn't in the starting; it's in the finishing. Anyone can get excited in the beginning. Anyone can talk a big game on day one. Real power is finishing what you said you would, even when it stops being fun, even when no one's watching.

Every time you leave something half-done, whether it's a goal, a plan, a workout, or a conversation, you train yourself to doubt your edge. That hesitation creeps into everything. Business. Discipline. Relationships. When you hesitate in one area, you bleed hesitation into all of them. When you build a pattern of finishing what seemed unachievable, you carve out trust. Self-trust is the most powerful asset a man can carry. Be the man who follows through. Not for applause. Not for perfection but because you said you would and watch the door of opportunities open for you.

Action:

1. Track Open Loops: Write down every unfinished task, promise, or project that remains outstanding. Personal, professional, and emotional. Be ruthless.

2. Rank by Weight: Which ones are draining the most energy? Handle those first. Light work avoids real work. Face the heavy ones.

3. Schedule Completion Time: Don't just "intend" to finish—block time. Set the alarm. Commit to a finished window as if your word were law.

4. Finish in Silence: No need to post or boast. The quiet finisher builds more power than the loud starter. Let your consistency speak.

5. Reward with Purpose, Not Distraction: When you complete, reward yourself with reflection or levelling up, not with numbing out. You're reinforcing power, not escaping effort.

November 7th

Show Up When You're Tired

It's easy to take action when you're rested, motivated, and everything is flowing smoothly. Real strength is revealed when your energy is drained, your mind is foggy, your body aches, and there's no spotlight. No applause. Just you and the decision: get it done or quit.

The masculine man doesn't wait for motivation. You move on command through owned discipline. Fatigue doesn't slow you; it sharpens you. Resistance doesn't stop you; it focuses you.

You don't need to crush every session, but you do need to train with intent. You don't need the perfect words, but you stay grounded in conflict. You don't feel inspired, but you deliver the work with excellence because you have a standard and a code.

Every time you show up tired, under pressure, or on the edge, you're raising the standard for who you are, both internally and externally. You're conditioning your nervous system to perform under stress, not just when conditions are perfect. You're building a version of yourself that doesn't rely on comfort, motivation, or mood to take action. You know that pushing through fatigue expands your capacity. Avoiding it drags you back to average. The man who keeps showing up when it's hard becomes the man who never doubts his strength because you've proven it in the moments that count.

Action:

1. Pick the one thing you've been avoiding because you're tired, uninspired, or drained.

2. Attack it. Not recklessly, but with discipline.

3. Adjust the pace, lower the reps, but finish. Don't let how you feel dictate who you are.

November 8th

Train Your Mind Like a Weapon

Powerful men are self-built through mental warfare, discipline, and daily sharpening of the one weapon: the mind. Your body can hit a wall. Status can fade, but your mind, when trained relentlessly, becomes your endless arsenal and your advantage on the battlefield.

Masculine dominance is the ability to outthink when others react—the man who trains his mind to play the long game while others chase the dopamine hit. You speak less because you're listening more, and when you do speak, it's with precision and commands attention.

Train your mind daily through solitude, breath, reflection, strategy, and observation. Challenge your thoughts, question your reactions, and refine your beliefs. Read, write, and review—study not just for knowledge but to understand your triggers, blind spots, and patterns. Be the man who knows your mind is untouchable because you control the one thing the world constantly tries to hijack.

Don't wait for a crisis to build mental strength. Prepare in advance. Control your inner world so nothing external can own you. That's how you become unshakable. That's how your mind becomes a weapon. Not recklessly but by ruthless precision.

Action:

1. Set aside 20 minutes to sit in silence. No distractions. Ask: "What thought patterns weaken me? What habits dull my edge?"

2. Write the answer. That's your next battlefield. Train there.

November 9th

Conquer One Vice at a Time

Every man carries a crutch, the quiet dependency that weakens your edge. It could be sugar, porn, constant distraction, validation-seeking, or the excuse you justify when no one's watching. Whatever you can't walk away from owns you.

Masculine mastery starts by reclaiming control, not all at once, but one vice at a time. You don't need to be perfect, but you need commitment. Every crutch you kill is a layer of mud removed, enhancing your power. It's one less thing draining your energy and time, one more step toward clarity, focus, and dominance.

The man ruled by impulse is predictable, and predictable men are easy to control. The man who denies the short-term hit for long-term strength becomes rare; rare men become unstoppable.

It's about self-respect. You don't quit out of shame. You quit because you're building something bigger. Keep stacking wins until there's nothing left that owns you but your mission.

Let Pain Refine You, Not Define You

Pain is not the enemy. It's your coach, and every hit, heartbreak, failure, and rejection carries a message and a lesson that makes most men flinch. They avoid it. They numb it. They allow pain to write their identity instead of sharpening their edge.

A masculine man doesn't let pain make him weaker; he welcomes it, making him stronger. You listen to the lesson despite the discomfort. You track the pattern, adjust the behaviour, adapt, and upgrade your baseline. Pain becomes the cue for the new level you're about to step into, not the chain that holds you back.

Emotional maturity and masculine evolution stop you from asking, "Why me?" and start asking, "What is this teaching me?"

When you respond with awareness instead of avoidance, every wound becomes wisdom, and every scar becomes a road map. The world doesn't need another man avoiding pain; it needs masculine men who master it.

November 11th

Practice Controlled Exposure

Power through controlled discomfort, over and over again. The masculine man doesn't wait for adversity to arrive; he meets it on his terms. Standing tall, calm, clear and ready. You introduce your system —body, mind, and breath — to the edge deliberately. Extreme exposure without intention is trauma. Exposure with intention is training.

Controlled exposure is a method for preparing your nervous system to cope with panic. It's about training your breath to remain steady in the face of stress. It's how your mind stops seeing a challenge as a threat and starts reading it as an opportunity.

Controlled exposure isn't just about tolerating discomfort; it's about commanding yourself through it. The man who trains for pressure, on purpose, becomes the man no pressure can break.

Action:

1. Cold Exposure: Ice Bath. Focus on breathing with no resistance. Start with 1 minute and gradually increase the time as needed. Train your nervous system to stay calm under pressure by stepping in without preparation and without acknowledging the discomfort. Go past the point where your mind tells you to get out, and when you do, step out calmly and composed.

2. Weekly Fear Reps: Identify one small thing that makes you hesitate, such as a challenging conversation, public speaking, or trying something new. Do it deliberately. Don't chase success, step into your strength.

3. Physical Intensity: Push past your previous training limits. One more round. One more sprint. Finish on an odd number. Don't stop when it burns; observe how you respond when it does.

4. Mental Stillness Under Stress: Sit in silence for 10 minutes immediately after a high-stress situation. Don't react, recalibrate.

5. Environmental Challenges: Change your routine environment weekly by taking an unfamiliar route, working in a new space, and training in a different outdoor location. You're learning adaptability.

November 12th

Embrace Boredom as Training

We've been conditioned to chase stimulation. To scroll. To fill every quiet gap with noise. A man who cannot sit with himself in silence is a man who doesn't yet own himself.

Boredom isn't the absence of action; it's the exposure of your inner chaos. When you run from boredom, you're not avoiding emptiness; you're avoiding yourself.

Masculine strength isn't just about action. It's about intention inside inaction. In the stillness, your patterns surface. Your wounds speak. Your truths rise. The man who learns to stay present without reaching for distraction begins to refine his edge from the inside out.

Boredom isn't a weakness. It's your next form of resistance training. The man who can sit in silence without needing to escape becomes immovable because you're no longer running from yourself, and no man is more powerful than the one who doesn't break into his thoughts.

Action:

1. Set a Timer for 15 Minutes of Nothing: No phone. No music. No journal. Just sit. Breathe. Observe your thoughts without reacting.

2. Name the Impulse: Every time you feel the itch to move, distract, or fidget, name it. "Avoidance." "Restlessness." "Fear." Labelling exposes the pattern and builds awareness.

3. Let Thoughts Pass Like Waves: You don't need to fight against your thoughts. Let them come. Let them pass without engaging in them.

4. Track the Resistance: Record any thoughts or feelings that arose after the session. What were you avoiding? What triggered discomfort?

5. Repeat every 3 Days for 30 Days: Make stillness a part of your training routine, just like weights or movement. Your ability to be still becomes your psychological weapon.

November 13th

Build Grit, Not Glamour

Grit isn't pretty. It doesn't trend. It doesn't give you dopamine hits or social media applause. It's early mornings when your bed feels better than your mission. It's pushing through reps when your body says stop. It's making disciplined decisions when comfort calls you to quit.

You don't build masculine strength by doing what looks good. You make it by doing what's necessary, over and over, especially when it's inconvenient. That quiet repetition, those unsexy standards, that invisible struggle, that's where true confidence and conviction come from. Not hype. Not hope. Hardened experience.

Grit makes you trust yourself because you've earned it. You've proven to yourself that when pressure comes, you hold your ground and get it done. That's unshakable. The masculine man doesn't crave attention. He craves the edge, and grit is the edge that endures.

November 14ᵗʰ

Track Your Weakness Like a Predator

The masculine man doesn't pretend. He observes. He stalks his flaws like prey, using them as a strategy. You don't rise by hiding from your cracks. You rise by tracking them, calling them out, and bleeding them dry of power with purpose. Your insecurity, temper, procrastination, and need for approval are each a leak in your system. Left unchecked, it becomes your ceiling. Hunted down, it becomes your fuel to remove your ceiling permanently.

You don't fear the parts of you that are unrefined; you confront them with intensity and presence. That self-awareness becomes your advantage in the arena of life. Cracks in your armour don't make you less of a man. Avoiding it does.

You don't become powerful by chance; you become powerful by choice, and that choice starts with the courage to face your shadows until they have no attachment to you.

Action:

1. Identify Your 3 Core Weaknesses: Write them down clearly. Not vague traits, specifics. "I scroll when I should build," "I avoid confrontation," "I don't finish what I start."

2. Name the Pattern: When and where do they appear? What triggers them? What do you usually do instead of addressing them?

3. Create a Strike Plan: One daily behaviour per weakness that directly attacks it.

   If you tend to procrastinate, set a 20-minute timer every morning to help you get started.

   Say "No" once a day when it's misaligned.

   If you avoid pain, Schedule cold exposure or a hard convo weekly.

4. Track the Kill Count: Journal your wins. Did the weakness win, or did you? Be honest. Progress is your scoreboard.

5. Reinforce with Reps: Precision + repetition = rewiring. Don't attack once and retreat. Recalibrate daily.

November 15th

Discipline > Motivation

Every man feels inspired when it's easy. Few act when it's cold, early, lonely, or inconvenient. That's the separator. That's the edge you have.

Discipline isn't about hype or the culture of hustle. It's about identity. A masculine man doesn't train because he feels like it; he trains because it's who he is. You don't lead, love, build, or push because it's convenient; you do it because it's coded into your DNA through repetition and resolve.

Discipline dictates your decisions, the ones you repeat when no one's watching. Every early wake-up, every extra rep, every time you say no to impulse, you lay another brick in the foundation of your unstoppable identity. Most men miss that discipline isn't emotionless; it's emotional mastery. You still feel tired, distracted, and triggered. You don't give in to it. You move through it.

Motivation is catching you on a good day when you'll feel like it. Discipline is becoming the man who does it because it's what you do.

November 16th

Remove Limiting Language to Unlock Relentless Action

You don't just train your body; you train your language because words shape reality. Most men put up walls before they even begin by calling it a grind, a struggle, a challenge, a sacrifice. These words inject resistance into your nervous system before a single move is made. They've already convinced themselves it will be hard, heavy, or painful, and that slows them down.

Even in everyday language, phrases like 'I'm too tired,' 'I've been too busy,' and 'I hope it's a safe flight' all carry doubt, fear, or limitation. The masculine man rewrites that script. When you drop the struggle story, your energy becomes focused, clear, and forward moving.

Approach what's ahead with the same precision and passion as a five-year-old boy playing to win, with no fear of consequence, no concern for opinions, just full action grounded in knowing. You don't hesitate; you attack and adjust as you move. That's not recklessness; it's unleashed power.

Words are frequency, and they prime your nervous system for action or avoidance. If you speak like it's going to be hard, it will be. If you act as if it's already done, your brain follows that command. Language is leadership, and you lead yourself first with the words you choose.

Action:

1. Eliminate Weak Language: Catch yourself saying hard, grind, sacrifice, tired, busy, try, hope, and replace them. Use precision, execute, own, present, locked in instead.

2. Speak as if your next move has already been made. Not "I'll try to work out," but "I train today because that's who I am."

3. Approach Everything Like a High-Stakes Mission: Stop Softening the Path. Remove the mental friction. Your edge is on the other side of language.

November 17th

Push Physical Limits Quarterly

Softness breeds apathy. Pushing your limits breeds growth. The masculine man doesn't need chaos to come knocking; you schedule it deliberately, with intent, on a quarterly basis. You know that the body holds the memory of what it has conquered, and your soul expands when it's tested.

Ultra-endurance runs. Martial arts immersion camps. Freediving courses. Long-distance hikes through remote terrain. A month of brutal training. A solo trek off-grid. These aren't hobbies; they're calibrations. Each one strips away excuses and reveals the truth: You either sharpen or you shrink.

Quarterly intensity resets your standard. It purges stagnation, renews focus, and humbles the ego while refining who you are when things get real. Prep 6 weeks out. Go all in. Reflect after. Repeat.

Action:

1. Q1: Choose an endurance challenge (50km run, City to City ride, multi-day hike).

2. Q2: Commit to a combat or skill-based immersion (Freediving course, Boxing intensive training and fighting).

3. Q3: Go solo (backpack wilderness trip, survival weekend, no phone, no support).

4. Q4: Tackle a full-body upgrade (train for a triathlon, Intense body transformation, or outdoor expedition).

November 18th

Don't Avoid Failure, Engineer It

If everything you do works or is a success, you're not playing big enough. You're managing risk, not building power. A masculine man doesn't just accept failure and lessons; you engineer them. You intentionally step into arenas where your success is minimal or regarded as impossible because you're not chasing comfort; you're seeking growth.

Every rep that breaks you. Every idea that doesn't pay off. Every moment where your plan falls apart is data. Failure is pressure testing your system. It reveals your edges, your ego, and your gaps in preparation, and once you see them, you can sharpen them. Weak men avoid failure to protect their image. Strong men seek to upgrade their reality. Learn. Recalibrate. Reload.

What it teaches:

1. Humility without collapse.
2. Adaptation without excuse.
3. Persistence without validation.

Information Doesn't Equal Power, Integration Does

Most men today hoard information like status symbols, bookshelves full, podcasts on repeat, and courses half-finished, but they never test it where it matters. They're addicted to learning but allergic to pressure. They mistake information for transformation. That's not mastery.

A masculine man understands that reading is preparation, not completion. True power comes when you apply that knowledge under tension, under pressure, when failure is a consequence. It's the moment when you're tired, overwhelmed, challenged, or uncertain, and you still move with precision using what you've learned. That's when knowledge becomes power.

You can read about breathwork, but until you're standing in confrontation and using it to regulate your state, you haven't integrated it. You can study negotiation tactics, but until you're in a room with six figures on the table and a ticking clock, you haven't earned the skill.

Men who never test their knowledge under fire remain stuck in theory. They sound intelligent but fold under pressure. Masculine wisdom expands through experience, not memorised in theory.

November 20th

Build Friction into Your Routine

Every day offers two choices: comfort or conditioning. Most unconsciously choose comfort; they automate weakness. High-level men understand that strength is sharpened by challenging moments, and those moments don't need to be dramatic. They need to be consistent.

Start with micro-decisions: Skip the elevator. Wake before the sun. Eat for fuel, not pleasure. Silence the phone. Delay the dopamine. Each one reclaims control from comfort. Each one trains your mind to obey your mission, not your mood.

When discomfort becomes familiar, fear loses its grip, and when you stop avoiding what's difficult, your standards rise automatically. Masculine growth isn't loud. It's in the quiet, gritty moments of chosen difficulty.

Action: (Daily)

1. Walk Instead of Drive: If it's under 20 minutes, use your legs. Train presence while moving.
2. Delay Gratification: When the urge to snack, scroll, or speak arises, pause for three deep breaths before acting.
3. Take the Harder Option: An extra set. One more rep. Every choice is sharpening you.

4. Sit in Silence: No phones. No music. 10 minutes a day. Let your thoughts surface. Watch them without judgment.

5. Reflect Every Night: Ask: "Where did I choose ease today? Where did I create strength?" Track it.

November 21st

Stop Negotiating with Your Standards

Standards are your inner architecture. They define the line between potential and performance. Most men treat them like suggestions. One tired day, and they bend. One distraction, and they dissolve. That's not power; that's permission to stay average.

Every time you negotiate with your standards, you dilute your discipline. You teach your mind that comfort wins, that your word means nothing. If your word doesn't lead you, no one else will follow it either. The edge isn't about doing more; it's about doing what you said, especially when it's inconvenient. You don't need to be in a good mood to stay on your mission; you show up because of your standards—no inner debate. No negotiating.

Action:

1. List Your Non-Negotiables: Choose 3 to 5 daily and weekly standards (e.g., 5:00 am wake-up, 60 minutes of training, no phone after 9:00 pm). These aren't goals. These are minimums.

2. Write the 'Why' Behind Each: Tie each standard to your identity. "I train daily because I lead myself before I lead others." Clarity builds commitment.

3. Track It Visibly: Use a wall chart or a dedicated app. Physically check off each standard every day. Let the streak sharpen your edge.

4. Add Consequences for Breaking One: If you break it, you will pay the price of 11 burpees and a cold plunge at 10 pm. Consequence builds discipline.

5. Reassess Monthly: Are your standards too low or too high?

November 22nd

Crave the Unknown

Certainty is comfortable, and comfort is decay in disguise. When everything is scripted and safe, there's no demand for adaptation. There's no reason to evolve. The unknown is the arena where warriors are born. It's where instinct replaces routine, presence replaces planning, and chaos reveals who you are without the armour.

The masculine edge lives in uncertainty. When you step into the unknown - a new business, a foreign environment, or a decision with no backup plan - your senses heighten. Your thinking is firing. Your leadership sharpens because there's no script, just you and the moment.

You grow by showing up in spaces where you don't have control and becoming the man who can command. Your power doesn't come from knowing the outcome; it comes from becoming a man who can face any outcome and adapt. That's where your masculine evolution accelerates because the version of you you've never met lives there, waiting to come out.

November 23rd

Challenge Your Body to Free Your Mind

Mental anguish is often a symptom of living in physical comfort. When your body is soft, your mind becomes loud. Doubt creeps in. Indecision grows. Insecurities stack up. Your thoughts scatter with no discipline. When you put your body through controlled stress, your focus locks in, your muscles shake, and your mind figures out how to keep going without breaking; that's when something primal happens.

You stop thinking and start being. Pain removes pretence. It forces you to be present. No past. No future. Just your breath. Just grit. Just you.

That's why you don't just train for aesthetics; you train for clarity, stillness, and presence under pressure because a challenged body produces a liberated mind.

The more you choose hard physical thresholds, the more doubt and mental chatter you clear. You begin to trust yourself, and you stop overanalysing. You think sharper, lead stronger, and feel fresher inside. The fastest path to inner peace is through outer discomfort.

Action: (45 mins)

1. Choose your threshold
2. Cold plunge
3. Intense hill sprint set
4. Heavy lifting under fatigue
5. Long-distance endurance session
6. Lock in presence: No music. No distractions. Just your breath and your movement.
7. Midpoint check-in: At your hardest point, ask: What am I afraid of right now? Face it. Don't let it distract you; move through it.
8. End with stillness: 5–10 minutes of seated meditation with a connected breath or walking in silence. Let your clarity land.

Surround Yourself with Men Who Level You Up

Your growth will eventually reach a ceiling by the standard of the men you keep close to. If your circle tolerates excuses, comfort, or mediocrity, you'll unconsciously do the same. You won't even notice you're stagnant because average looks normal when you're surrounded by it.

Surround yourself with men who demand more, and everything changes. Their presence will expose your blind spots. Their standards will make you feel uncomfortable. Their wins will challenge your self-image, and that's the point.

Masculine growth requires friction. Steel sharpens steel. You need to feel slightly behind in the right room; that's how you know you're growing. Stepping out of your comfort zone and having trust in the men guiding you to the next level. Find the right communities, ones built on values, change, and accountability. Don't just belong somewhere because it's in trend. Belong where the baseline is power, where mediocrity doesn't survive. Where your future self already exists.

Find a mentor. Not a cheerleader but a proven man who has been through the fire and emerged stronger. A man who commands respect without noise. Someone who sees your next evolution, even when you can't.

Action:

1. Audit your five closest male influences: Do they challenge your thinking? Do they elevate your habits? Would you trade places with any of them in one key area of life?

2. Leave one stagnant circle this month: Be honest: where are you coasting because it's comfortable?

3. Join a high-level environment: Men's group, elite mastermind, or aligned brotherhood with structure, leadership, and pressure.

4. Find a mentor or coach: Don't choose someone popular. Pick who lives the life you want with strength, integrity, and results. Commit to learning, not just knowledge, but embodiment.

November 25th

Comfort and Complacency Make You Replaceable

Comfort kills progress. Complacency buries potential. For the masculine man, these two forces are the silent destroyers of growth, both in business and in life. When you become too comfortable with your results, income, reputation, or routine, you tend to become complacent. You stop taking the strategic risks that stretch your capacity and redefine your position.

In business, being comfortable means, you're no longer hunting. You're no longer sharpening your message, expanding your reach, or backing yourself under pressure. You've settled. Men who settle often get replaced, overlooked for deals, passed over for leadership, and eventually forgotten in the market. Complacency is weakness dressed in routine. It feels safe, but it's silently eroding your masculine edge.

As a high-level masculine man, you don't just maintain; you evolve. You move with calculated force, knowing that your reputation, wealth, and power are built on the fire of uncomfortable decisions. If you're not adapting, testing yourself, and pushing the line of what you can own, you're already becoming irrelevant.

Your presence in the business world, just like in life, must be undeniable. Not because you're loud but because you're always in motion, constantly refining, and always ready. That's what builds the kind of dominance that can't be ignored or replaced.

November 26th

Live Getting Busy, Not Anxious

The masculine man understands the weight of time, not as pressure, but as presence. You're not frantic, rushed, or chasing the clock. You know that life doesn't wait, and neither should you. So, get busy - not just in motion, but on your mission, your purpose, and your legacy. Not to prove but to progress. You don't panic at the unknown but are grounded in the only thing that matters, which is what you do now.

Plan as if you've another hundred years ahead, but live as if your number could be up tomorrow. That's not fear-based; that's power in momentum, clarity in purpose and self-trust to achieve your legacy.

When you live with integrity, morals, and purpose, your actions hold weight. You don't have to rush, but you do have to move. Most men are waiting for the perfect time or perfect conditions. The masculine man builds while others hesitate. You read. You train. You initiate. Every day is an opportunity to extract more from yourself, acquire new knowledge, cultivate greater strength, and discover a deeper purpose. Not someday. Everyday

You'll never regret learning more or sharpening your skills, but not achieving your mission, purpose, or legacy, while you had more in the tank to give, will sit with you until the end. Get busy getting it done now.

November 27th

Study What Threatens You

Finance, negotiation, conflict resolution, and managing pressure aren't just skills; they're essential tools. If they intimidate you, you've already given them power. If you avoid them, they grow in the shadows. When you study them relentlessly, train under real-time experiences, and expose yourself to them repeatedly, you build dominance in the very space that once made you hesitate.

You learn to breathe when you want to snap. You negotiate when your voice can shake. You stay still when every emotion is screaming to run. That's absolute masculine control. That's embodied confidence, not the kind you fake online, the kind you carry in your nervous system, calm, precise, and untouchable.

Turn what once broke you into something you now command.

Action:

1. Identify one area that still owns you: What do you avoid, delay, or fear exposure in?
2. Make it your next mission: Study it as if your life depends on it. Practice it until you embody it.
3. Track your edge: Every week, put yourself in a scenario where you test this weakness under pressure.

November 28th

Earn Your Rest Through Effort

True masculine rest is earned, not assumed. It's not the soft escape from pressure. It's the reward after pressure has been met, moved through, and conquered with force, clarity, and commitment.

In the modern world, too many men confuse laziness with self-care. They take breaks without building momentum. They celebrate small wins as if they've won the war, but they haven't even left the training ground.

The masculine man doesn't operate like that. You calibrate your rest to the weight of your effort. You know when you've pushed your edge and when you're cheating yourself. You don't celebrate too soon, as you understand every achievement is not the finish line; it's just a milestone. A checkpoint. A signal that the next level now opens. If you waste your energy on ego-driven celebrations, you lose momentum. You release the drive you've just built.

That doesn't mean celebrating; it means knowing when you've earned the celebration. Know the level of the win. Know the energy it costs. Know how much you still have to give. A king doesn't throw a parade every time he swings the sword; he celebrates after he has won the battle and the kingdom is secure.

Action:

1. Measure Your Output Honestly: Ask, 'Did I truly push today?' Did I face resistance, make real moves, or coast?

   If the answer is soft, delay rest and earn it. Your nervous system knows when you're lying.

2. Set Milestone Thresholds: Create specific markers for when you can rest or celebrate. Example: No downtime until the project draft is delivered. There is no reward until 5 days of clean execution are logged.

3. Design Your Rest Ritual with Intention: Choose a recovery that recharges you positively and still supports your forward momentum and purpose.

4. Use Momentum to Forecast the Next Climb: Before you rest, define the next challenge.

November 29th

Let Challenges Reveal
Who You Are

You don't meet the real man when you are in times of ease. You meet him when the room gets heavy, when the air tightens, when your plans fall apart, and nobody's coming to save you. In that moment, when everything feels like it might collapse, the mask drops. The rehearsed confidence fades. The ego can't hold up. Only your truth remains. That's the moment that separates boys from men, pretenders from leaders, and noise from presence.

Tests don't build you; they reveal who you are. It doesn't care about your image, your Instagram persona, or the smooth words you speak when nothing's at stake. It wants your essence. It digs into your soul and asks: What's left when everything is stripped away?

In those moments, you don't need to know all the answers. You don't need the perfect playbook. You need to be grounded. It's in those silent grounding moments that your inner legend is born, not the public story, not the headline, but the internal shift where you finally know who you are. It's raw. It's real.

You don't train for this moment by reading more. You train for it by leaning in and experiencing it.

The masculine man doesn't chase the applause; he chases the edge. It's at the edge, and he meets the man he was always born to be. The one who doesn't need to fake power because he is power. Quiet. Unshakable. Whether it's self-belief or a high power you believe in, you know you are here for greatness, and nothing is going to stop you.

November 30th

Step In. Don't Look Back

There comes a point where thinking becomes the enemy. Where planning, analysing, and perfecting are just dressed-up forms of fear. You've trained. You've prepared. You've sharpened your tools, and now it's time to get it done.

The modern masculine man doesn't wait for perfect conditions; You create movement. You step into the unknown not with hesitation but with conviction. Not because you're sure of the outcome but because you trust who you're becoming through the process. That's the shift from needing guarantees to embodying a knowing.

When the fear and doubt creep in, when your mind starts whispering all the "what ifs", you remind it: "I don't chase comfort. I master evolution," because everything you want is behind that door, and you step through ready for action.

The Ultimate Masculine Man

Integrate Everything. Live as a Modern Warrior, Philosopher, King

This month is where it all converges: strength, purpose, power, presence, leadership, and love. You've been sharpening every edge; now it's time to live it fully. As The Ultimate Masculine Man, you don't just master areas of life; you integrate them into one relentless, refined identity.

You are not just a man who trains, builds, and conquers. You are a man who leads with depth, who protects with clarity, who governs himself like a kingdom. The modern warrior isn't wild, you are aware. You don't chase chaos; you channel it. You don't speak of mastery; you live it, moment by moment, decision by decision.

This month marks the activation of your total embodiment. No fragmentation. No contradiction. Just full-spectrum masculine presence. The man who can sit in silence, then lead under pressure. The man who can destroy when necessary and nurture when needed. The man who can live as a protector, provider, savage, and safe space, all in one breath.

You're not building anymore. You're becoming, and from here on out, there is no turning back because you've seen what you are capable of. Now, it's time to embody it. Daily. Decisively. Unapologetically.

"Be the man who commands without noise, conquers without doubt, and lives with nothing held back."

December 1st

Know Yourself, Brutally

The foundation of true masculine power is not brute force or blind ambition; it is ruthless self-awareness. To know yourself brutally means you stop living in an illusion. You no longer confuse confidence with ego, distraction with purpose, or motion with progress. You become the observer of your mind, the architect of your character, and the interrogator of your own story. You don't just know your traits; you understand the truth behind why you behave, react, withdraw, chase, or dominate.

A high-level, masculine man studies himself like a strategist reviews a battlefield. Every unconscious pattern is a hidden opponent. Every unprocessed wound is a liability, and every unresolved fear is an invisible leash limiting his reach. Until you see these, they own you.

Start with your emotional blueprint. When do you shut down? When do you lash out? What situations cause you to betray your standards, to manipulate, or to withdraw? These aren't random; they're echoes of past pain, unmet needs, and stories you're still carrying from childhood or past failures. Brutal self-awareness means you stop blaming the world for what you haven't healed in yourself. You track your emotional reactions back to the root and confront them without flinching.

Next, study your coping mechanisms. Where do you go when things get hard, porn, food, fantasy, overwork, fake positivity? These aren't bad in isolation, but they become programmed traps used to escape your edge. Masculine men don't just welcome growth; they examine what's blocking it. Self-sabotage always hides in the shadows of unexamined comfort.

Then, identify your gifts and blind spots. Knowing yourself isn't just about exposing wounds; it's also about owning your power. What are you naturally sharp at? What do people consistently look to you for? What environments unlock your best self? Too many men focus on fixing what's wrong and forget to amplify what's right. Your purpose is encoded in your patterns, but it only emerges when you slow down and take the time to observe.

True masculine self-awareness also means becoming aware of the stories you've outgrown. Perhaps you're still acting like the boy who needs approval. Maybe you're still chasing achievements to prove something to a father who never gave praise. None of these stories are the truth; they're survival codes, applicable once in your past, and now they're outdated in light of who you are today.

To be a brutally self-aware man is to strip your identity down to its raw core and then rebuild it consciously. You make the unconscious conscious. You stop reacting and start choosing. You become the kind of man who can stand still, alone, in silence, and know exactly who he is, what he believes, what he'll fight for, and where he's going.

Once you know yourself fully, no one can manipulate you, and no challenge can break you.

It's not self-help. It's self-command, and from there, you build everything.

December 2nd

Define Your Code

As a masculine man, you are not defined by how loud you are, how much you lift, or how much attention you get. You're defined by the invisible law you live by, your code. A blueprint for how you move, how you speak, what you accept, and what you walk away from.

Without a code, you're a drifter, swayed by trends, emotions, and weak influences. With one, you're a mountain, unmoved, unshaken, and unmistakably clear.

Your code is built through self-awareness, brutal reflection, pressure, pain, failure, and wins that come with a cost. It must be written in stone, not sand. If it changes to match your mood or social circle, it's not a code. It's a costume.

This code becomes your:

- Standard — how you carry yourself.
- Shield — what protects your peace.
- Weapon — what makes you trusted and influential?
- Compass — how you find direction when everything feels unclear.

You don't invent your code. You uncover it by asking:

- What values do I hold even if they cost me?
- What behaviours violate my integrity?
- What do I tolerate that silently erodes my power?

When pressure rises, your code tells you how to move. When your emotions flare, your code recalibrates your response. When temptation knocks, your code answers with clarity.

Examples of a Masculine Code:

1. I speak the truth, even when my voice shakes.
2. I do not act from fear.
3. I protect the peace, mine and hers.
4. I train daily, mind, body, and purpose.
5. I never negotiate with disrespect.
6. I finish what I start.
7. I lead, even when it's hard.
8. I always show up for those who depend on me.

December 3rd

Recalibrate Your Nervous System

The Masculine man is no longer about brute reaction; it's about refined regulation. It begins not with a mindset but with nervous system control. Your nervous system is the gateway between your primal instincts and your conscious precision. When your nervous system is tested by fear, overstimulation, or unresolved trauma, you'll lash out, freeze, or retreat. You'll confuse emotion for intuition, and you'll make choices based on survival, not strategy.

At the core of masculine presence is autonomic mastery, the ability to shift from sympathetic (fight, flight, freeze) to parasympathetic (calm, control, command) at will. The man who breathes through pressure doesn't just survive it; you own it. You slow time and sharpen your thoughts. You neutralise threats, both perceived and real, and become the calm eye in the centre of the storm.

Recalibrating the nervous system begins with breath. The breath is the only part of your autonomic system you can consciously control, and when mastered, it becomes the manual override to panic, anger, overwhelm, and shutdown.

Train your breath, and you train your state.

- Deep nasal breathing stimulates the vagus nerve, your body's calm command centre.
- Breath holds increase CO_2 tolerance, meaning you become more efficient under stress.
- Long exhales regulate heart rate variability, the pulse of resilience and emotional control.

The masculine man uses breath not just to survive a moment but to dominate it. When others feel fear, you exhale more slowly. When your woman spirals emotionally, you don't meet her in panic; you become the anchor she didn't even know she needed.

Beyond breath, nervous system mastery includes:

- Stillness practice to expand your emotional container.
- Sensory integration to process trauma somatically, not just mentally.
- Movement training to re-pattern how your body stores and releases stress.

A regulated nervous system also creates deeper intimacy. Recalibrating your nervous system is not optional. It is the foundation of tactical masculinity. When your body stays calm, your mind becomes lethal.

December 4th

Grounded

To be grounded as a masculine man is not a personality trait; it's a physiological state, a trained behaviour, and a spiritual position in the world. It means you are anchored in your body, present in the now, and immovable by fear, urgency, or external chaos. The grounded man remains calm and precise in the face of tension.

Biologically, grounding is the nervous system's signal of safety and regulation. When you're grounded, your breath is deep and paced, your muscles are relaxed but ready, and your eyes hold attention without force. It's about your thoughts, emotions, breath, and biology being in alignment, and because of that, your external world begins to organise around your presence.

Psychologically, being grounded means narratives, emotional hijacks, or reactive patterns do not sweep you up. You can hold multiple perspectives without losing yours. You don't argue for validation. You don't explain when silence says more. You respond to pressure with discernment, not drama. A grounded man knows who he is, and because of that, you can walk through a jungle and still make clear decisions. Your presence is medicine, your energy is fresh, and your intentions are precise.

Spiritually, grounding is the deep-rooted knowing that life is happening for you, not to you. That you are not separate from the rhythms of the earth, the cycles of challenge and ease, or the laws of cause and effect. A grounded man honours timing. You don't rush because others are panicking. You don't chase trends, clout, or hollow victories. You listen to his intuition, trust your gut feeling, and move in alignment with something far greater than the news cycle or emotional drama.

To become grounded, a man must train his awareness. You must slow down your breath under pressure and lower your voice when provoked. You must learn to feel his feet on the ground, keep your gaze steady, and regulate your tone so it transmits clarity instead of confusion.

A grounded man doesn't just survive modern life; you master it. While others are reactive, addicted to stimulation, and pulled by every emotional wave and mental backwash, you remain centred. Real masculine strength in today's world is rare, which makes you unstoppable.

December 5th

Disciplined

Discipline is not willpower. It is not motivation. It is the embodiment of a standard that does not bend under pressure. In the masculine man, discipline is a form of identity. It is not something you turn on when you feel inspired; it is who you are, especially when you don't feel like it. Your day doesn't run on emotions or convenience; it runs on clarity, integrity, and execution. When others hesitate, you move. When others talk about change, you're already getting it done.

To be disciplined is to have a structure that frees you, not cages you. The modern masculine man understands that freedom without discipline lacks direction disguised as potential. You know that every great warrior, artist, or leader has one thing in common. Sacred repetition. Boundaries that channel energy into mastery. Discipline is the masculine man's daily ritual to your vision, and you earn it through relentless consistency.

The undisciplined man chases short-term dopamine: the scroll, the hit, the comfort. As a disciplined man, you train your system to crave progress, not pleasure. You delay gratification, building momentum with every rep, every action, and every business decision. You understand that the actual payoff is not just in the results; it's in who you become by choosing the hard path again and again. This rewiring is measurable. It's neuroplasticity activated by repetition under tension.

When you say, "I will", and follow through, you prove to yourself that your word holds weight. In a world where most men break promises to themselves before breakfast, this becomes rare and powerful. The disciplined man does not allow comfort to dilute his character. You create alignment between what you say, what you believe, and how you act. This alignment becomes magnetic. It signals trust in others and stability in relationships and business.

A disciplined man does not waste hours on drama, gossip, or idle distractions because they understand that life is a war and every moment is a valuable resource. Your calendar is a battlefield of priorities. Your routine is armour against chaos. You move with purpose because you know the mission matters. Whether you're training your body, building an empire, raising a family, or sharpening your mind, it's all sacred.

The masculine man who is disciplined becomes unstoppable, not because you have more talent or resources, but because you are dependable to yourself. What needs to be done is done every day until you become the embodiment of your word.

December 6th

Visionary

The masculine man who embodies vision is not operating from impulse; he's operating from insight. You read patterns others miss and see not just what is but what could be. While the average man reacts to what's in front of him, the visionary masculine man operates from foresight. You map your moves, understand ripple effects, and position yourself and others to win.

Being a visionary means operating with precision in a world obsessed with speed. It's playing chess while others play checkers. The masculine visionary doesn't chase instant wins; you create sustainable empires. You don't get lured into distractions or petty battles because you know every decision either builds the mission or slows it down. You value time as the highest currency, and you spend it on outcomes, not what-ifs. It's about structuring your life in alignment with a higher direction, guided by purpose, values, and conviction.

A masculine man also masters the invisible, intuition, pattern recognition, and emotional intelligence. Neuroscience backs this: the brain's prefrontal cortex, responsible for long-term planning, is most active in calm, intentional states. That's why the visionary man must first master presence. Without a presence, you're reacting. Without discipline, your ideas are delusions. When presence and discipline are combined with strategic thought, the results are strong leadership. You train your awareness to scan for signals: market shifts, emotional currents, and spiritual direction. Your mind isn't cluttered because you filter information ruthlessly. You ask: Does this align with my direction or distract from it?

The masculine man then reverse engineers that vision into actionable systems. You build the bridge between where you're going, what's now and what's next. You develop rituals, train skills, and surround yourself with others who challenge your thinking and expand your edge. A true visionary empowers allies and communicates with clarity so others can carry the mission forward.

December 7th

Move from scarcity to abundance

To move from scarcity to abundance is to make the psychological, emotional, and spiritual shift from chasing to attracting. This transformation sits at the core of true masculine power. Most men unknowingly operate from a scarcity of time, love, money, and worth. It is embedded in how they speak, how they negotiate, and how they show up in relationships. It sounds like urgency, desperation, and overcompensation. Performing for validation, attaching identity to status, and bending values for temporary gain. Scarcity is not just about what's missing in your life; it's about the unconscious belief that there's not enough and that you are not enough.

The sovereign man understands he is the source, not the beggar. You don't wait for permission, validation, or opportunity; you create it. It's the embodiment of ownership over your mind, energy, time, and choices, and from this place, you stop chasing. You stop needing everything outside yourself to complete you. You become magnetic. People feel your clarity, your presence, and your non-attachment, and they lean in because abundance, unlike dominance, doesn't push; it draws in without effort.

Gratitude is the weapon that gets you there. Genuine gratitude is a practised awareness of abundance in the now. It's being able to look at your current reality, however difficult, and extract power from it. Neurologically, gratitude increases dopamine and serotonin, the chemicals of confidence, connection, and grounded energy. It rewires your brain away from a threat-response (scarcity) mindset into one of resilience and optimism.

When you are in fear about your income, your relationship, and your status, your decisions become reactive. You hoard energy, grasp at control, and choke opportunity. When you're grounded in gratitude, you begin to trust your state again. You don't just want to win; you bring value, direction, and decisiveness to the room because that's who you are. The energy of "I need this deal" becomes "This is what I offer. It's either aligned, or it isn't." That subtle shift changes everything.

You walk away from disrespect. You stop explaining your worth; you let your life be the proof. You don't enter a room to dominate. You enter grounded, aware, and connected to yourself, and that presence commands respect.

To move from scarcity to abundance is the death of the desperate boy and the birth of the grounded king.

December 8th

Relentlessly Accountable

Accountability is the cornerstone of true masculinity. To be relentlessly accountable means that a man lives in a world where your word is law, where excuses have no oxygen, and where outcomes, good or bad, are traced back to you without self-judgment. A man who is relentlessly accountable reclaims full ownership of his life. You understand that nothing changes until you do, and nothing improves unless you're willing to hold the mirror and do the work.

In a culture of victimhood and avoidance, accountability is a rebellion. It's the masculine man's refusal to outsource responsibility for his emotions, results, relationships, or destiny. You don't point fingers when life gets hard; you recalibrate your actions. When someone wrongs you, you confront it, but you don't collapse into helplessness. You examine where your boundaries were unclear and your awareness low. That self-examination doesn't weaken you; it makes you stronger, more precise, and far more dangerous in the arena of life.

Once a man removes blame, you become untouchable. You can no longer be manipulated by failure, stalled by betrayal, or broken by circumstance. You understand that even if it wasn't your fault, it's still your responsibility to respond with power, clarity, and forward motion.

This level of ownership permeates every aspect of life: business, fitness, finances, brotherhood, and intimacy. In leadership, the relentlessly accountable man never says, "That wasn't my doing." You say, "I'll figure it out." In relationships, you don't gaslight, ghost, or guilt-trip; you communicate with clarity, and you own your emotional patterns. If you break a trust, you name it. If you break her heart, you make space for the impact.

Relentless accountability shifts the nervous system from helplessness (fight/flight/freeze) to empowerment (prefrontal leadership). You no longer react. You respond. You identify, adapt, and move forward with purpose.

Stop hoping life will change; instead, become the one who makes the change. Stop demanding others show up better, and you show them how.

December 9ᵗʰ

Sharpen Emotional Command

A masculine man with emotional command isn't empty of feeling; you're in full possession of it. Many confuse self-command with suppression, assuming masculinity means never feeling sadness, anger, or fear. Numbness isn't strength, it's shutdown. Likewise, volatility isn't power; it's a loss of self-control. True masculine power lies in the ability to feel everything without being ruled by anything.

To sharpen emotional command means to become the container, not the chaos. It's conscious regulation and the ability to observe emotional spikes without reacting impulsively. When you develop this internal leadership, you become the calm in any storm, not because you avoid emotion but because you've chosen to step into your feelings and learnt to channel them.

A man must learn how to shift from a reactive state (sympathetic fight-or-flight) to a grounded state (parasympathetic rest-and-respond) through breath, presence, and awareness.

Emotionally immature men perform in one of two extremes: suppression or outburst. Both are forms of self-abandonment. The man who suppresses avoids the discomfort of expression. The man who explodes avoids the discipline of presence. You don't guilt-trip, shut down, weaponise your pain, or seek to control. You bring emotional safety. You know the difference between emotional presence and emotional projection. You speak directly and listen actively, and you see the way you express emotions teaches your woman how safe she can be, not just with you but with herself.

December 10th

Build Physical Presence

A masculine man does not separate mind from body; you understand they are integrated and linked. Physical presence is not vanity. It's not about aesthetics or performance for the approval of others. It is about discipline, integrity, and self-mastery.

The masculine body is not just something to look at; it is something to trust. It must be dependable under pressure, capable in battle, and transcend resilience through pain. Whether you're in the gym or on a mountain, in the boardroom or stepping into an emotional conflict, your body broadcasts your readiness to act, and readiness is the difference between potential and power.

Training daily isn't about being addicted to the gym; it's about honouring the responsibility of having a body that is ready for anything. When you train, you're not just building muscle. You're building identity. You're learning how to push through pain in a controlled way without losing focus. That process flows into every other domain of your life: how you lead, how you protect, and how you show up for others.

A weak body leads to a scattered mind. Suppose you cannot hold the tension of a heavy barbell or tolerate the pain of lactic acid. How will you hold the tension of a failing relationship or a multi-million-dollar negotiation? When you become physically capable, your nervous system recalibrates, and you feel safer, and you don't avoid hard things; you seek them.

When the world gets soft, the masculine man gets sharp. You move weights because you want to feel your edge. You run hills because you want to hear your breath's rhythm under pressure. You practice fighting styles because you must be able to protect yourself and others. The day may come when it's required, and when that day comes, there will be no time to prepare; you will be ready.

Your body is the one possession you carry everywhere, into every room, every challenge, every season of life. When you honour your body, you become ready for everything.

December 11th

Protective Without Possession

The mature masculine man does not confuse protection with ownership. You know that true strength is not about domination or surveillance but about presence, stability, and accountability. To be protective without possession is to become a guardian, not a captor. It is the ability to stand between your loved ones and harm while still allowing them the autonomy to live, evolve, and express themselves without manipulation or suppression. This is not a weakness. It is restraint governed by wisdom.

When you have done your inner work, you don't protect yourself out of fear; you protect yourself from a place of purpose. You protect because your presence is grounded and capable. This kind of man will walk your partner home every night, not because you don't trust her, but because you value her. You will scan the room when they walk in, not to control where she looks or who she speaks to, but to ensure the environment remains safe. You will support her growth and allow her to stumble and find her way, stronger knowing you are there. You will challenge her, not diminish her. You know that being masculine doesn't mean overshadowing; it means amplifying. Your strength becomes her sanctuary.

Masculine protection is also not loud or performative. It is quiet, alert, and ever ready. The protector trains, physically, emotionally, and spiritually, not to posture but to prepare. You prepare to de-escalate a confrontation, to hold space during emotional storms, to step in if danger appears, and to stay calm when darkness occurs. Your calm energy must say, "Nothing happens to you while I'm here."

December 12th

Speak with Precision, Not Performance

Speaking with precision means your communication is intentional, not impulsive. You don't talk to impress. You speak to influence. You don't need the spotlight, applause, or emotional validation because your value is not externalised. The man who has mastered the art of masculine speech knows that his words should cut through noise, not contribute to it.

Your words carry no power if your mind is cluttered with indecision, emotionally reactive, or if you hold unprocessed wounds. If your speech is vague, your mission will lack direction. When your mind is sharp, your values are defined, and your words become razor-sharp reflections of your inner command.

You learn to eliminate filler, fluff, justification, and weak disclaimers. You don't say, "I think maybe…" — you say, "This is where I stand." You don't say, "I feel…, or I believe…" You speak directly with an undeniable knowing. You don't use five sentences when one will do. Masculine speech is concise, grounded, and unshakable.

The masculine voice is not loud; it's clear. A man who raises his voice to prove a point is already losing the battle. The more grounded your nervous system, the steadier your voice becomes.

You don't react with sharpness or sarcasm; you respond with certainty. Not monotone or lack of expression but the resonance of your voice that reflects the weight of your intent.

To speak precisely also means to listen deeply. You don't interrupt to prove intellect; you listen to extract meaning. You listen with your lips slightly open and not tightly closed, waiting to talk. You're studying. You're sensing patterns, energy, and inconsistencies.

In a world of talkers, be a man of few deliberate, powerful words. Speak less. Speak with precision.

December 13ᵗʰ

Quietly Dangerous

The masculine man who embodies quiet danger is a rare paradox that commands respect. You are not loud. You are not reactive. You don't need to boast about your skills or intimidate with bravado. It is internal, earned, sharpened, and ready. You walk into a room, and people feel a calm weight—a presence. Your danger is not a threat; it's a promise: you can handle anything.

To be quietly dangerous means, you've trained in silence. You've put in the reps —physically, mentally, and emotionally —not for applause but to be prepared. You've stepped into the ring when others avoided it. You've broken under pressure and rebuilt without witnesses. You've tested your edge in solitude when there was no one to impress. You've done the hard work of learning how to stay composed in crisis, navigate your emotions without letting them spill over, and maintain your composure when others lose theirs.

The masculine man who is quietly dangerous has refined his skills in combat, business, emotional control, and strategy. You're not looking for fights, but if conflict comes, you don't back down.

Your woman feels safe in your arms because you're grounded in your body. Your business partners listen because you speak from knowing. Your enemies don't challenge you because they can feel, without needing proof, that you're not the one to underestimate.

Choosing to rise when broken, to master skillsets instead of relying on brute force, and to walk away from the noise because you don't waste energy proving what's already proven.

You are dangerous because you are disciplined. You are trusted and respected because you have done what most men avoid. That's what it means to be quietly dangerous. You don't just look strong; you are the storm they never saw coming.

December 14th

Seek Tests Like Oxygen

To be a masculine man in the modern world is not to seek comfort, applause, or ease; it is to seek tests the way your lungs seek air. Tests are not something you endure; they are what you pursue. Only in the pursuit of adversity do you meet your authentic self, raw and unbreakable. The masculine man doesn't grow by reading about strength. You become it through immersion in discomfort, repetition under resistance, and presence in pressure.

Choosing the hard path is a strategy. When you voluntarily put yourself on the battlefield, you control the transformation. You dictate the pace of growth, the direction of pressure, and the identity that emerges. You don't sit back and wait for the universe to test you; you create your proving grounds. You run into the wilderness, sign up for the fight, wake up when it's dark, and do what most men postpone. You know that the longer you avoid difficulty, the weaker you become, and the weaker you become, the more you'll be ruled by the world around you.

Learning new skills when your ego wants to avoid being a beginner. Standing in front of failure and not shrinking from it. These are not just acts of resilience; they are rituals of transformation. They rewire your nervous system, they sharpen your mind, and they elevate your spirit.

A man who seeks tests becomes unshakable. While others panic, you breathe. While others hide, you step forward. Your default becomes forward motion. You train you're your body and mind to respond to pressure with presence. It is about seeing life not as something to be endured but as something to be experienced in every way.

December 15th

Strategic Thinker

To embody the role of a strategic thinker as a masculine man is to rise above the reactive mindset that dominates weak men and mediocre leadership. It's not about outsmarting others in manipulative ways; it's about seeing deeper, planning further, and thinking beyond the surface. As a strategic man, you don't simply respond to what's in front of you; you observe the terrain, see the ripple effect of every decision, and act from an elevated vantage point. This kind of thinking is learned through stillness, reflection, and pattern recognition.

You study psychology, game theory, military strategy, negotiation, biology, and power dynamics, not for vanity but for mastery. You understand that every area of life, love, money, war, and peace, is a battlefield of decisions. You're not surprised when conflict shows up; you predicted it three steps ago, and you have already made your move and peace with it.

The masculine man balances foresight with internal composure. You regulate your nervous system so that when the pressure rises, you don't default to impulse. You slow down internally to make faster decisions externally. Clarity is a weapon, and it's a weapon earned through the practice of intentional breath and inner stillness.

A strategic man understands that some moments require immediate action while others require a long game with surgical precision. You see human behaviour not as random but as a cycle — predictable when studied, mastered when understood.

Most men live on reaction, driven by triggers and fleeting desires. The strategic masculine man lives on precision. You stay quiet, observe, plan, and you strike when it matters. You position yourself for the opportunity, not out of luck, but because you've created leverage over time, and when others panic, you're already in motion.

You don't play small games. You're building a legacy quietly, intentionally, and relentlessly.

December 16th

Turn Pain into Power

When others are numb, collapse, or break down, you lean in. You study the wound, honour its message, and turn it into strategic wisdom. You know, the man who can master pain becomes the most dangerous force in any room because you are unbreakable from within.

Whether it comes from heartbreak, betrayal, financial collapse, family dysfunction, abandonment, failure, rejection, or self-sabotage, you don't run from it. You don't drown it with distractions, substances, or noise. You breathe into it. You allow it to expose the unconscious patterns, the generational cycles, and the emotional residues that most men spend their lives trying to avoid. You identify it and refine it into insight, conviction, and inner steel.

Pain is not just emotional; it resides in the nervous system, in posture, in breath, and in how a person speaks and holds space. You don't pretend your past doesn't matter. You acknowledge every part of your story, even the darkest chapters, and you extract goodness from what it taught you.

You are the man who understands that everything is feedback. The loss of a relationship shows you where he abandoned your integrity. The betrayal by a friend shows you where you ignored the red flags. The collapse of a business reveals where you failed to lead or prepare. You treat every bruise as a blueprint, every failure as an experience, and every fall as a training ground for your next level of evolution.

Life will break every man at some point, but very few rise with more clarity, compassion, integrity, and command. You don't just survive; you emerge with a clear mission, an open heart, and a deep presence of a warrior.

December 17th

Calm Under Fire

In the presence of chaos, most men revert to survival mode. Emotions flare, the breath shortens, tunnel vision sets in, voices rise, and clarity dissolves. As a masculine man, you're built differently. Your breath slows down. Your voice stays. Your decisions become more deliberate. You read the battlefield, see the patterns, and act from a place of grounded clarity.

This level of composure regulates the autonomic nervous system. When the sympathetic system (fight or flight) is triggered, most men either explode with aggression or freeze in indecision. You've trained yourself to shift into parasympathetic dominance on command, activating calm, clarity, and strategic thinking in real-time. Activating this comes through deep breathwork, stress exposure training, and neuro-regulation practices that are practised daily and programmed into your baseline response.

In love, this shows up when your woman brings an emotional storm. You hold space, listen with still eyes, hold her with grounded arms, and speak from calm truth. In business, this shows up in high-stakes negotiations, financial pressure, and high-speed pivots. You don't beg, chase, or fold; you play from clarity and let others react.

You are not calm because life is easy. You are relaxed because you've become the kind of man whose storms cannot shake; you are the storm and the stillness in one.

December 18th

Deeply Respectful

To be deeply respectful as a masculine man is not to bend, appease, or submit. It is to walk through the world with honour, a rare trait in a culture that confuses loudness for strength and dominance for power.

A man who cannot respect himself will unconsciously seek to take from others what he hasn't cultivated within. He'll posture, manipulate, interrupt, or disrespect boundaries because, internally, he hasn't formed his own. The deeply respectful man has already fought that battle. You've looked at your shame. You've reconciled with your past. You've earned your respect through discipline, truth-telling, physical training, emotional mastery, and spiritual grounding.

You now walk tall not to impress but because of your mission, your purpose, and your legacy.

You honour the feminine, not in the performative way of weak men seeking approval, but in the solid way of a protector who sees the beauty, mystery, power, and life itself in her feminine expression. You see her as sacred, powerful, and worthy of protection, not control. Whether it's your lover, daughter, sister, or colleague, your respect is evident in how you listen, how you speak, and how you stand beside her.

You respect the earth, not as a trend, but as a warrior does a battlefield that feeds your energy. You train in the cold, the mountains, the heat, and the ocean, not just for fitness but because nature is your temple. As a deeply respectful man, you don't seek to conquer nature; you desire to sync with it. You know that disrespecting the environment is another form of disrespecting yourself. You lean into your primal source and draw wisdom from it.

You respect your mission, your purpose, your legacy, and the reason for rising when others cannot. The deeply respectful man doesn't betray his mission to chase trends or attention. You move with intention, knowing that time is limited, and your calling is non-negotiable.

Respect is evident in minor details, such as maintaining eye contact, good posture, firm handshakes, active listening without interruption, and respecting personal space. You are not the "nice guy." You are kind with a backbone and move with direction.

The deeply respectful masculine man is the rare combination of power and grace. You can destroy, but you choose to build. You can dominate, but you decide to lead. You can take, but you choose to serve, and that choice is made daily, moment by moment, with words, presence, and energy.

December 19th

Lead with Integrity in all Arenas

Integrity isn't just a noble idea for the masculine man; it is the root system of your entire existence. True masculine integrity means a seamless intention between thought, word, and action. It means that what you say, what you do, and what you believe are all aligned.

A masculine man understands that every promise you make becomes a piece of your foundation.

You don't overcommit to please, and you don't underdeliver to protect your ego. You only say what you are ready to build, lift, or die for. Owning your failures, your missteps, your truth, and in a world addicted to image, integrity is a rebellion, a return to substance over show.

In business, this means deals are built not just on profit but on principle. It means your handshake means more than a signature, and you negotiate with clarity and fairness. You know that trust is the ultimate currency, and reputation is the actual return on investment.

In brotherhood, integrity means you don't speak differently behind a man's back than you do to his face. It means you hold your brothers accountable, not with ego, but with honour. You speak the truth when it's uncomfortable, and you receive the truth without defensiveness.

In the bedroom, integrity is the difference between manipulation and connection. It means you lead sexually with presence, not performance. You don't seduce them with false promises for your gratification. You don't disappear after intimacy or wield emotional leverage. You show up, not just with your body, but with your whole self. You listen. You honour. He sees it as a sacred exchange, where her surrender is a response to the trust you build, not a result of games played.

To lead with integrity in all arenas means you live as one whole man. Who you are when no one is watching is the same man who shows up on the stage, in the boardroom, in the bedroom, and the storm.

The masculine man is not just respected for what you achieve but for how you achieve it, and that alignment becomes your unshakable kingdom.

December 20th

Unapologetically Bold

You are unapologetically bold, not because you're loud, not because you seek attention, and not because you're trying to impress. You are bold because you live in alignment, and alignment creates certainty. It is the quiet authority of knowing who you are, what your values are, and where you're heading. You don't ask for permission to take up space in the world. Your presence is grounded, not inflated. Your words are deliberate, not desperate, and when you speak, it's not to dominate; it's to direct.

Boldness, in its purest masculine form, is the willingness to walk into discomfort without flinching. You walk through the world without needing to look over your shoulder to hide or for approval. Your worth is internal through discipline, deep self-respect, and facing your demons. You have become a man who can lead, not because you are better than others, but because you no longer betray yourself.

The masculine man is precise with his words, calculated in his energy, and clear with his boundaries. When you draw a line, it is not a threat; it's your standard. People don't respect you because you demand it; they respect you because you walk with a presence that says: "I've done the work. I know what I tolerate, and I stand by it."

You hold space for your woman's emotions without losing your centre. You say "no" when needed. You choose clarity over comfort, even when it's hard. You initiate difficult conversations, and you protect her peace by protecting your integrity.

You are bold because you are grounded, and being grounded means you've become immovable, not from stubbornness, but from a deep knowing that you've faced your fears. You move with conviction, and you don't just live differently; you change lives by walking into them.

December 21ˢᵗ

Harmonise Masculine and Feminine Within

A truly masculine man is not just the embodiment of dominance, aggression, or strength. You are a fully integrated man who has done the deep inner work to recognise, honour, and harmonise both your masculine and feminine energies.

Masculine energy is the sword: purpose-driven, structured, disciplined, and penetrative in intention. It's the calm in chaos, the silence in storms, the still presence that grounds a room and a woman alike. Without the feminine energy, the part of you that is intuitive, emotional, receptive, fluid, and creative, your masculinity loses depth, and you won't connect. You may succeed, but you'll feel hollow. You may lead, but no one will want to follow.

On the other hand, a man who is all emotion, all intuition, all sensitivity but lacks the structure to hold it becomes scattered, unstable, and often resentful. Integration means you are both the container and the current. You can lead a woman without controlling her, listen to her without losing your edge, and love her without abandoning yourself.

This harmony isn't about being "soft." It's about being whole. The untrained man is reactive, either collapsing into his emotions or repressing them entirely. The integrated man can hold grief in one hand and action in the other. You can stand in front of a room, grounded and composed, while still being attuned to the emotional undercurrent of silence. You don't fear intimacy, nor do you sacrifice your mission for it. You are both fire and water, depending on what the moment calls for.

The feminine in your partner will not open to a man who is emotionally unavailable or spiritually disconnected. She also won't trust a man who is unstable, needy, or constantly in a state of emotional collapse. When you integrate your masculine and feminine, you become the man she can lean into, not because you're perfect, but because you are solid. She senses your depth and your ability to lead, not just in direction but also in emotional intelligence.

To harmonise these energies, you must do the deep work. Shadow work to confront where your feminine energy has been wounded, where you've learned to suppress, to disconnect, to dominate instead of listen. Breathwork, embodiment practices, and nervous system recalibrations aren't spiritual buzzwords; they're practical tools to anchor presence and unlock wisdom.

You become the modern warrior, philosopher, and king. Not just because you win battles but because you know when to hold when to guide when to listen, and when to strike.

December 22nd

Expand from Presence, Not Pressure

You don't measure your worth by how much pressure you can endure. You don't buy into the outdated myth that the more you grind, suffer, or sacrifice, the more masculine you become. True masculine evolution begins the moment a man stops chasing the world from a place of lack and starts expanding from the ground of presence. Not reactive. Not impulsive. Tuned in. Aligned. Focused.

It's the state where your nervous system is regulated, your awareness is sharp, and your actions are deliberate. A man in presence is not hurried, even in urgency. You know when to act, when to hold, when to strike, and when to wait because you listen to the subtleties within your body, not the noise outside.

A man who expands from presence operates on a different frequency. Your power doesn't spike; it sustains. You have trained your body and mind to stay grounded in high-stakes situations, to return to your breath when urgency peaks, and to read the situation before reacting to it. Your very being becomes directional. Strategic. Magnetic.

This presence translates into every domain of your life. In business, you don't overtalk or oversell; you own the room with your calm presence. You listen before you speak, observe before you act, and speak only when your words carry weight. Every move has a reason, and that reason is rooted in your long-term vision, not emotional survival.

To live from presence requires inner training. Breathwork is essential. You must learn to regulate your system under stress to reset your baseline from a state of fight-or-flight to one of calm command. Stillness is your practice field. Solitude becomes your teacher. You must learn to sit in discomfort, in silence, in uncertainty, without reaching for distractions or compulsions. The man who can keep his breath steady while others unravel is the one who leads. The man who can sit in uncertainty without forcing an outcome is the one who sees clearly.

Expansion is no longer a matter of grinding more hours or stacking more effort; it's energetic conservation and focused precision.

December 23rd

Choose Love with Leadership

To choose love with leadership is to rise above the juvenile archetypes of the needy lover, the manipulative seducer, or the emotionless alpha image. It is the embodiment of the modern masculine man who understands that love is not weakness and leadership is not dominance. It is a conscious integration of emotional intelligence, sexual connection, grounded presence, and unshakable standards. A man who chooses to love with leadership knows that attraction is not something you chase; it's something you align with. You don't perform for validation or contort your truth to gain attention. You hold your frame and move with purpose, and in doing so, you become the force that draws in a high-quality partner, not out of need, but out of frequency.

Begging, chasing, or playing games are tactics of a man disconnected from his core. They come from fear of abandonment, insecurity, or a distorted view of love as conquest. As a masculine man, you don't beg for love because you are already full within yourself. You have cultivated solitude into strength, turned pain into power, and you know that your self-worth is not dependent on another's approval. You have developed the confidence to walk alone if needed, and that's why people want to walk with you. Your love isn't an escape from emptiness. It is an extension of your completeness.

Leadership in love means guiding the relationship with clarity, stability, and strength. It means being the one who navigates emotional storms without pushback, initiates difficult conversations with presence, and creates the space where the feminine can feel safe to soften, expand, and express. You don't expect her to carry the burden of emotional regulation, financial planning, or future vision; you bring those gifts first. You're not just a protector in the physical sense; You're a protector of emotional space, spiritual alignment, and relational direction.

Holding space isn't passive; it's a powerful act of masculine containment. It means you stay grounded when your partner is emotional, remain curious when she's closed off, offer support when she's scared, and stay strong when she tests your boundaries. You don't collapse under her tests or compete with her expression. You remain solid, aware, and attuned, not because you're trying to "win" her emotions but because you're leading from depth.

As a masculine man, you create a shared vision, build structure, and initiate rituals. You cultivate intimacy not just through words or sex but through attention, touch, time, and direction. When you master this, you no longer fear love, resent the feminine, or hide behind detachment. You claim the throne in your own heart, and from that place, you create a kingdom where love thrives with strength, direction, connection, and devotion.

December 24th

Focused on Impact Over Image

When you have evolved and live with devotion to your purpose, not addicted to your image, you don't live for applause, vanity, or social validation. You are focused on impact because you understand that lasting influence is achieved through consistent action, personal integrity, and results that ripple long after your voice is quiet. In a culture obsessed with the optics of masculinity, highlight reels, performance posturing, and curated personas, you stand as a reminder that real power does not require display. It changes lives in silence.

You don't waste energy trying to be perceived a certain way. You know the difference between being respected and being seen. While others shout for attention, you refine your craft, deepen your character, and lead from the front lines. You don't flex; you build, not for followers or fame, but because your legacy demands more. Legacy growth loves repetition when no one is watching. Every decision goes through an internal process: "Will this create change? Will this matter when I'm gone?"

To live this way demands discipline. It requires resisting shortcuts and temporary gratification. It means choosing the unsexy work over the glamorous gimmicks. You are not interested in selling a lifestyle. You are here to live a life worth studying, not based on likes, comments, or approval metrics. Your metrics are growth, transformation, loyalty, and outcomes, and you do it through presence, example, and execution. You're not the man who posts about doing the work; you're the man doing the work.

Being focused on impact means you don't allow your emotional energy to be wasted trying to be validated by strangers; self-containment makes you more effective.

This way of life isn't for everyone. It requires you to kill your ego daily, to face your insecurities without hiding behind an image, and to build something bigger than yourself.

December 25th

Build Systems, Not Just a Hustle

The masculine man who seeks mastery in his life, whether in business, purpose, relationships, or legacy, must evolve beyond raw effort and embrace intelligent structure. Hustle, for all its glorified grind and adrenaline-fueled momentum, is a short-term play. It may work when you're hungry, unknown, or proving yourself, but a hustle is not scalable. Hustle ties your results to how hard you can push in a single day. The masculine man understands that if your vision is to outlive you, you must shift from being the engine to becoming the engineer. That means building more refined systems.

A system is the difference between a man who builds a machine that works only when he does and a man who creates something that runs with or without him. When you build systems, you begin to extract yourself from being the bottleneck in your empire. You increase output while decreasing burnout. It's the evolution from warrior to king, where the kingdom runs on structure, not excess energy output.

In business, this means documenting your processes, delegating your weaknesses, and installing clear feedback loops. You don't just "do marketing"; you have a marketing system. You don't just "sell"; you have a sales process that educates, qualifies, closes, and retains. You don't just post when you feel inspired; you have a content machine that runs consistently because it's connected to a more profound message, a clear offer, and a proven conversion path.

You build systems in your fitness, finances, mental state, and relationships. You don't work out "when you feel like it"; you create a training protocol. You don't try to save money randomly; you have investment frameworks and income flow that support your wealth creation.

This level of customisation requires a mindset shift. You stop seeing yourself as the hero of the story and start becoming the builder of the structure that creates heroes. You stop solving the same problems over and over. You make a system that eliminates the problem.

Every man who wants to stop being consumed by a single mission must eventually step into this higher order of masculine embodiment to grow his purpose and create a solid legacy. Real power is not how much you can do in a day; it's how much you can build that continues to do long after you stop.

December 26th

Free

Freedom is not the absence of responsibility. It is not avoiding commitments, running from pressure, or living detached from consequences. It is the result of ownership, ownership of yourself, ownership of your decisions, and ownership of your power. The free man is not the one who escapes struggle but the one who walks into it with conviction.

To be free as a masculine man means your emotional state is not at the mercy of others. It means no one can manipulate you with guilt, rejection, or temptation because you have done the brutal work of shadow integration. You've faced the parts of yourself that once ran the show from the background: the boy who sought validation, the addict who needed to escape, the pleaser who feared disapproval, the perfectionist who needed to earn his worth. You've looked them in the eye, and you've outgrown them. It's neurological and behavioural transformation, cultivated through repetition, reflection, and real-world consequences.

You choose discipline not because you're a slave to rules but because you're a master of focus. You know who you are, and you accept the responsibility of being that man, even when it costs you comfort, followers, or approval.

You are not a man who fears losing a woman because you do not lose yourself. You hold space, not control. You offer love, not dependency. You choose a connection from wholeness, not need. The woman who stands beside you is selected, not as a need to validate your self-worth.

You have created leverage through skill, through systems, as a thought leader. You don't sell your soul for short-term gain. Your currency is value, your word is law, and because of that, you can walk into any room with calm command.

You're free because you no longer betray yourself to be liked, needed, or understood. The ultimate masculine man is not unbreakable, not perfect, but grounded in who you are, what you build, and why you breathe.

Train Your Environment to Reflect Your Standards

As a masculine man, you do not live reactively, letting your environment mould you without resistance. Instead, you train your environment the same way you train your body and mind: deliberately, with precision, and with unshakable intent. You know that everything around you —the space you wake up in, the people you interact with, the sounds you hear, and the conversations you engage in— either supports or sabotages your current mission.

To live in power, you must shape your domain to align with your standards. That means eliminating noise, visible and energetic, and replacing it with cues that keep your value at the top of your mind. An empty room with weights in the corner is a training ground. A desk with order is a war table. Books with depth are tools—a kitchen fuels performance. The environment becomes a reflection of who you are and a constant reminder of who you're becoming.

You do not keep company with those who tolerate mediocrity, gossip, or emotional instability. You surround yourself with men of direction, women of integrity, and mentors who sharpen your edge. You know energy is contagious, and if someone's presence lowers your frequency or weakens your mental state, you remove it.

Your external environment reflects your internal boundaries, priorities, and vision. If your environment is chaotic, it's likely because your mind is undisciplined. To elevate your life, you must first elevate your space and shape your surroundings until they sharpen you.

December 28th

Integrate Pain into Your Identity, Not Your Story

To integrate pain into your identity is to extract its lesson, sharpen your self-awareness through it, and reinforce your foundation with the truth it taught you. The pain is no longer something that happens to you; it becomes something now embedded within you, fuelling your decisions, instincts, and clarity. You stop telling the same story, seeking validation for your suffering, and instead let the experience refine your standards, your vision, and your ability to hold others.

This level of integration requires ruthless honesty and responsibility. You must be willing to examine the role you played, the illusions you held, and the weaknesses that were exposed. When you carry integrated pain, you don't speak from theory; you speak from experience. That's why your words carry weight that cuts through.

There's a difference between being in pain and being shaped by it. Most men stay stuck in the story, looping through old wounds, defining themselves by trauma, staying emotionally reactive and energetically stuck. The masculine man says, "This happened. It hurt. It exposed me. Now it strengthens me." You don't use it to justify being less; you use it to become more. Your heart is deeper, not because you have no wounds, but because you know how to transform your pain into love.

The masculine man is not the one who had it easy; you are the one who has faced adversity, transcended resilience, and the story behind it, and integrated it into your grounding.

December 29th

Master the Inner Dialogue, Become Your Commander

The battlefield of the masculine man is first within his mind. Before you can lead others, you must lead yourself, and that begins with mastering the mental backwash and the inner critic. Most men's internal dialogue is a loop of self-doubt, over-analysis, fear, and excuses. It sabotages their action before they even begin. The masculine man doesn't entertain the noise.

To master your inner dialogue, monitor it closely. It's not about "positive thinking"; that's surface-level. It's about recognising the tone, patterns, and impact of your internal language. Are you affirming weakness or activating strength? Are you hesitating with 'what ifs' or executing with 'what now'? The masculine man doesn't allow passive language in his mind. You don't say, "I can't," "Maybe," or "I'm not ready." You delete that from your operating system. Your inner voice is sharp, direct, and focused on progress.

You don't need a coach yelling at you, a crowd cheering for you, or even a reward to motivate you. You are the coach, mentor, and the force driving your thoughts and actions. You hear your internal resistance, and you override it. When your body says "stop," your mind says, "one more." When your emotions say "quit," your inner coach says, "Warm-ups over, let's get started." You discipline your thoughts like you would your muscles through consistent training, repetition, and feedback loops that reinforce power.

When your internal world is stable, decisive, and aligned, your external world follows. You don't waste energy battling doubt. You don't second-guess your action. Every great warrior, leader, and builder train their inner voice like a weapon.

December 30th

Embody the Mission Until You Become It

For the masculine man, the mission is not a concept; it's an internal identity. It is not something you visit when it's convenient or something you turn on when you feel like it. It is in your breath, your decisions, your movement, and in your silence—a man who "wants to find purpose" and the man who has become his purpose. One is playing at life, the other is life in motion.

You do not require permission or wait for signs, support, or applause. The mission drives you the way the heart pumps blood; it's automatic, necessary, and constant. Your discipline is not sourced from fleeting emotions but from deep internal alignment. The work, the training, the sacrifice, it's not a cost; it's a vow you made to something bigger.

Your rest is strategic, nutrition is fuel, and relationships are either aligned or released.

It's about living in a way that ensures every action feeds momentum instead of stealing it. The masculine man is not interested in dabbling. You don't dilute his edge or tiptoe around with scattered energy. You are surgical in how you spend your minutes because every minute is an investment in your long game.

When you get knocked down, and you will, you don't need motivation to rise and get moving again. The mission reminds you why you started, why you bleed for it, and why you must continue.

December 31st

Live With Your Legacy in Mind

The masculine man who embodies his legacy doesn't simply strive to succeed in the present; he engineers the future. Your vision extends decades beyond your own life. You understand that every decision, every word, and every behaviour is casting a ripple that will outlive you. Legacy is a system of alignment between who you are, what you do, and what will remain when you're no longer here.

You see time differently. You move with a long-term vision but get busy doing it now. You don't waste energy chasing applause or trend-driven success because you know those things evaporate. Your daily habits are not just about discipline for yourself; they are demonstrations for those watching silently, especially any man seeking a model of what's possible.

Living with legacy in mind means you train not just to be strong but to teach strength. You build wealth not just to spend but to empower others. You create not just for profit but to leave behind tools, wisdom, and frameworks that elevate humanity. You don't separate your personal life from your mission; you integrate both under a single standard.

When challenges arise, you don't just think about how to survive them; you ask, "What will this teach the next generation?" This level of thinking doesn't slow you down; it sharpens and elevates your energy.

Legacy is built in silence, not in the noise of social media or the applause of crowds. It's the discipline of your early mornings. It's how you show up for others when no one is watching.

A legacy-driven man doesn't fear death; you prepare for it by living fully and experiencing all you can now. You document your wisdom. You mentor intentionally, and you create assets that grow while you sleep. You make every moment count, not because you're obsessed with time running out, but because you know that time is the currency of impact. You don't just ask, "What do I want?" You ask, "What will endure because I was here?"

www.ingramcontent.com/pod-product-compliance
Lightning Source LLC
Chambersburg PA
CBHW040931050426
42334CB00059B/3004

*9 7 8 0 6 4 8 4 3 5 1 5 0 *